Yoga

IN THE
SHAMBHAVA
TRADITION

613.7046 D491
Devananda, Omkari, Swami.
Yoga in the Shambhava
tradition

MID-CONTINENT PUBLIC LIBRARY
Colbern Road Branch
1000 N.E. Colbern Road
Lee's Summit, MO 64086 **CR**

D0869362

WITHDRAWN
FROM THE RECORDS OF THE
MID-CONTINENT PUBLIC LIBRARY

Swami
Omkari
Devananda

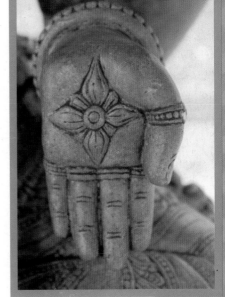

Healthy Living Publications
Summertown, Tennessee

© 2009 Swami Omkari Devananda
Photographs by Bob Carter
Paintings by Faith Stone

Cover design by Warren Jefferson

Interior design by Warren Jefferson, Gwynelle Dismukes, and Cord Slatton

All rights reserved. No portion of this book may be reproduced by any means whatsoever, except for brief quotations in reviews, without written permission from the publisher.

Published in the United States by
Healthy Living Publications
a div. of Book Publishing Company
P.O. Box 99
Summertown, TN 38483
1-888-260-8458

Printed in Hong Kong

ISBN-13 978-1-57067-199-9

ISBN-10 1-57067-199-0

15 14 13 12 11 10 09   9 8 7 6 5 4 3 2 1

Library of Congress Cataloging-in-Publication Data
Devananda, Omkari, Swami.
  Yoga in the Shambhava tradition / Swami Omkari Devananda.
      p. cm.
  Includes bibliographical references and index.
  ISBN 978-1-57067-199-9
  1. Hatha yoga. I. Title.

  RA781.7.D483 2009
  613.7′046--dc22

                    2008050294

Book Publishing Co. is a member of Green Press Initiative. We chose to print this title on paper with postconsumer recycled content and processed without chlorine, which saved the following natural resources:

- 38 trees
- 4,239 lbs. of solid waste
- 32,601 gallons of water
- 10,528 lbs. of greenhouse gases
- 70 million BTU's

BOOK
PUBLISHING
COMPANY

For more information visit www.greenpressinitiative.org. Savings calculations thanks to the Environmental Defense Paper Calculator at www.papercalculator.org.

Contents

Preface

MID-CONTINENT PUBLIC LIBRARY
Colbern Road Branch
1000 N.E. Colbern Road
Lee's Summit, MO 64086 **CR**

MID-CONTINENT PUBLIC LIBRARY
3 0000 13119200 1

HATHA YOGA IMPROVES THE HEALTH of every bodily system. It improves circulation and digestion, and strengthens the nervous and respiratory systems. Practiced regularly, it reduces stress and rejuvenates the body. It promotes clarity and awareness, and also improves memory. Hatha yoga is for everyone, for people of all ages and backgrounds. It is a physical discipline that improves well-being for both men and women. It is considered just one branch of yogic practices that also includes yama (guidelines for social conduct), niyama (guidelines for personal conduct), pranayama (breathing exercises), concentration (disciplining the mind), meditation (focusing on divine nature), drawing the senses within (pratyahara), and experiencing the state of realization (samadhi). For many, hatha yoga is an easy way to begin the process of opening within, and everyone, even the experienced practitioner, can benefit from some simple daily stretching.

To maximize the benefits from your practice, here are general precautions:

- Bathe and wear clean, comfortable yoga clothes.
- Practice on an empty stomach.
- Warm up first using simple stretches (see Chapter 6, pages 196-209). Add the Staff of Brahma (pages 74-75) and Sun Salutations (pages 76-79) to thoroughly prepare for the postures.
- Morning is best for practice, but you can practice anytime.
- Yoga is noncompetitive. Don't overdo it.
- Practice poses in conjunction with steady, regular breathing.
- When possible, learn from a teacher first and then practice at home.
- Avoid inverted poses during menstruation and if you have headaches; high blood pressure; or head, neck, or spine injuries. Check with a physician if in doubt.
- Practice variations as needed.
- Use common sense as a guide.
- Practice for fifteen minutes a day or longer, working with each pose for approximately one to two minutes.

Acknowledgments

THIS BOOK IS A COMPILATION of teachings that have been part of the Shambhava School of Yoga for years and thus represents the energy and effort of many individuals. I would like to extend my gratitude to those who contributed to writing, editing, graphics, and photography, and to those who teach and practice yoga in our school.

Special thanks to: H. H. Rishi Mahamandaleshwar Sri Shambhavananda, who founded our school; Faith Stone, for her love of sacred art and for her wisdom in the book *Rudi and the Green Apple;* Bob Carter, for his expertise in photography and cover designs; Swami Kripananda, for her graceful writing of the introduction and philosophy, help with photography, and guidance; Mukti Miller, for her tireless editing and good nature; and Satyam Ehinger, for his willingness to serve, and his assistance with the photography.

Also special thanks to the yoga models: Ram Best, Sara Bowman, Durgama Brook, Jyoti Fontaine, Karyn Karlson, Narayani Levine, Chandra Mazzeo, Mukti Miller, Chandra Supnet, Janabai Tull, and Maitreya Wood.

Also thanks to all the dedicated yogis at Shoshoni Yoga Retreat whose support made it possible for me to work on this book. I offer my deepest gratitude to Sri Shambhavananda, who continues to inspire and amaze us all.

Swami Omkari Devananda
Shoshoni Yoga Retreat

How to Use this Book

SINCE YOGA PRACTICE BENEFITS EVERYONE, find the category that best describes you and your needs, and begin your practice based on the recommendations. You will find hatha yoga sequences, meditation exercises, breathing exercises, and daily gratitude practices in each chapter. You may also wish to scan from cover to cover in order to choose what is most helpful to you.

Hatha yoga beginners:

- See Chapter 1 (pages 24-85) and Chapter 6 (pages 196-209).
- Progress to the other chapters when you feel ready for additional postures.

Hatha yoga practitioners:

- Try everything from Chapter 1 through Chapter 6.
- Be creative; choose a pose you haven't done and work on it.
- Practice with a friend to try postures you haven't done.
- Try all the Home Practice Sequences and then create your own.

Hatha yoga teachers:

- Add meditations, breathing exercises, and new poses to your classes.
- Flip through the book for inspiration and ideas.
- Try all the Home Practice Sequences to add new fuel to your teaching.

Meditators:

- Prepare for meditation by practicing the leg and hip stretches (pages 202-205), the Staff of Brahma (pages 74-75), and Sun Salutations (pages 76-79).
- Practice the Natural Breath Meditation (page 118).
- Practice the Heart Meditation (page 146).
- Practice combining mantra with meditation (see Chapter 1, page 83, and Chapter 4, page 174).

Those with busy lives:

- Practice the gratitude exercises at the start of each chapter.

🐚 Practice the breathing exercises when you have a break in your day.

🐚 Choose three favorite poses to work on when you can't attend a class.

Those who wish to relax:

🐚 Try the Home Practice Sequence (Chapter 6, page 209) to rejuvenate.

Those in recovery:

🐚 See Chapter 1 (pages 24-85) and Chapter 6 (pages 196-209) for gentle, nurturing stretches.

🐚 Practice the Heart Meditation (page 146) for ten minutes each day, morning and evening.

🐚 Practice the Basic Tension Release Practice (page 146) for at least five minutes each day.

Those who wish to use yoga for conditioning:

🐚 Practice the Sun Salutations (pages 76-79) and the Moon Salutation (pages 80-81).

🐚 Choose any pose and maintain the posture for up to two minutes.

🐚 Increase your daily posture practice to one hour.

🐚 Strengthen your mind with daily meditations (see Chapters 2, 3, and 4).

Those who have insomnia:

🐚 Practice the Leg and Hip Stretch Series (pages 202-205).

🐚 Practice the Bridge Pose (page 64), Shoulderstand (page 70), Simple Fish (page 65), and Wind Reliever (page 48) before sleep.

🐚 Practice five minutes of the Basic Tension Release Practice (page 146) before sleep.

🐚 Slowly practice the Full Yogic Breath (page 174) up to ten times as you fall asleep.

🐚 Practice repeating your favorite mantra until you fall asleep.

Those who wish to augment this book:

🐚 A variety of DVDs are available through the Shoshoni Yoga Retreat; please check the Shoshoni bookstore at www.shoshoni.org.

Ganesha Invocation

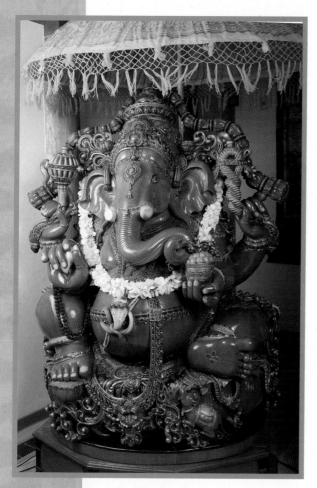

Ganesha

GANESHA is the name of one of the most beloved of all Hindu deities. His form is that of a round-bellied human with the head (and sometimes multiple faces) of an elephant. The elephant head is said to represent wisdom, understanding, and discrimination. The name Ganesha means "lord of the multitudes." This represents his role as one who oversees access to all forms of energy, removing obstacles, and opening doors for us. It is Ganesha whom we invoke when undertaking new ventures, or when we simply need help and understanding from the higher realms.

Ganesha is often invoked at the beginning of a trip, class, or new venture to help remove obstacles in our path. His mantra is used to invoke his blessing:

Om gam Ganeshaya namah.

The Spiritual Purpose of
Hatha Yoga

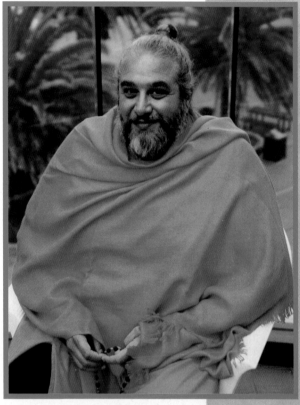

H.H. Rishi Mahamandaleshwar Sri Shambhavananda, Founder of the Shambhava School of Yoga

THE TRUE PURPOSE of hatha yoga is to refine the nervous system and to prepare the physical body to withstand the rigors of a higher level of spiritual work. It does have the side effects and benefits that people in our society often seek. It brings suppleness, strength, and flexibility that other exercise methods can't offer. But it is very seldom mentioned that hatha yoga was created for a spiritual purpose. One of those spiritual purposes is to provide a method to sit in meditation correctly for long periods of time.

These asanas were created for a higher spiritual purpose to help you in your spiritual evolution. Hatha yoga helps you bring your awareness inside. It helps you gain control over the flow of energy in your body. It teaches you to feel the pranic forces moving through your body and to feel the effect this flow has on your nervous system. As you become more attuned to your nervous system through the correct use of breath and motion and posture, you start to discover that there are energy centers known as chakras that are connected to your nervous system. The chakras hold information from your past lives, information about this present life, information about diseases that may manifest at some point, as well as information about the imbalances you suffer from on an emotional, physical, and mental level. Thus hatha yoga is a very powerful tool for inner development as well as a method for improving your physical health.

-Rishi Mahamandaleshwar Sri Shambhavananda, *A Seat by the Fire*

9

Introduction to the
Shambhava School of Yoga

THE SHAMBHAVA SCHOOL OF YOGA is named for the founder, Sri Shambhavananda, who is a modern master of kundalini meditation. He teaches by example that we can all attain spiritual liberation no matter what our lifestyle or personal circumstances. He teaches that we can use all of the situations of our life as an arena to fulfill and resolve our karma, and evolve spiritually. Sri Shambhavananda demonstrates through living example that opening our hearts and serving life requires only a deep wish to grow spiritually, along with the courage and willingness to make a commitment to our practice.

He deeply believes and teaches that the material and spiritual development that he has experienced over the last thirty years is a manifestation of his constant connection to the universal flow of energy. The creative potential that his first guru, Swami Rudrananda, unlocked so long ago flows strongly through Shambhavananda and draws creativity out of everything and everyone he comes in contact with. Individuals with latent talent find their talent spontaneously unfolding, abandoned properties develop into places of pilgrimage for yogis around the world, and children develop into mature and responsible members of society with a keen interest in spiritual development.

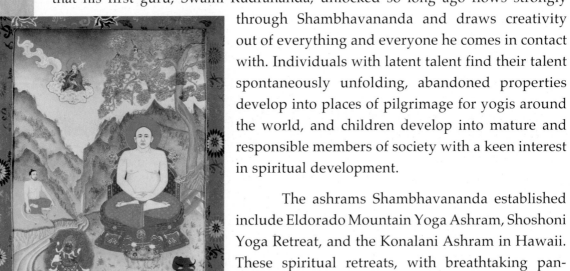

Swami Rudrananda

The ashrams Shambhavananda established include Eldorado Mountain Yoga Ashram, Shoshoni Yoga Retreat, and the Konalani Ashram in Hawaii. These spiritual retreats, with breathtaking panoramic views, have become the focal point of the spiritual path for a large and varied group of people from a variety of backgrounds.

Sri Shambhavananda began his sadhana (spiritual practice) in his early twenties, when he met Swami Rudrananda (known as Rudi) at Indiana University. Rudi was giving a lecture one evening, and one of Shambhavananda's friends invited him to come. He describes that experience as the turning point in his life—he says that Rudi literally "blew his mind." It seemed as though everything Rudi said that evening was directed right at him, as if Rudi could read his mind. He was trying to hide in his seat, but felt as if he were completely exposed. Many students describe the experience of being in their guru's presence this way. They feel as if they are naked—there is nothing they can hide. This is often a sign.

Shortly after this lecture, Shambhavananda went to see Rudi at his ashram, where he was initiated into the practice of kundalini meditation. His connection to this practice was deep and profound. This was due in part to the power and energy of the practice, but also because of the unlocked potential in Sri Shambhavananda.

Recognizing his extraordinary potential, Rudi initiated him into teaching kundalini meditation. He started an ashram and taught under Rudi's guidance and direction. Then, within only two years of meeting Shambhavananda, Rudi took mahasamadhi (great liberation). Mahasamadhi is when enlightened beings leave their physical bodies. Because they have realized the goal of human existence, this is considered to be a time for celebration. They have fulfilled all of their karmic obligations and are free to merge with Universal Consciousness.

Shambhavananda used the practices that Rudi gave him and taught them wholeheartedly for a number of years before meeting Rudi's former teacher, Swami Muktananda, at a meditation program in Florida. During darshan (being in the presence of a saint), Muktananda acknowledged him as "having very good shakti." Swami Muktananda treated him like a long lost son, showering him with love. Shambhavananda says that when he went in and sat with Muktananda, his heart burst open. He likes to say he got his PhD from Muktananda. While studying with Muktananda, he was given the name Shambhavananda and initiated into the Saraswati order of swamis. The name Shambhavananda means "bliss of the natural state of being that dwells within us as the Inner Self."

In the philosophy of Kashmir Saivism (a branch of Hinduism), Shambhava is one of the highest upayas, or paths to enlightenment. The Shambhava upaya is described as the sudden emergence or recognition of divine consciousness by a mere hint from the guru. This is the path of a very evolved soul. Just as a ripe piece of fruit requires only a slight breeze for it to fall from the tree, very mature seekers require only that they meet someone who is immersed in the bliss of the Self to realize their own liberation. Muktananda recognized a quality and capacity in him that earned him the distinguished title of Sri Shambhavananda.

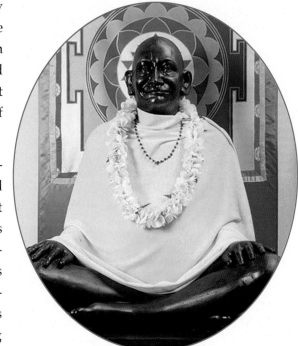

Murthi of Bhagavan Nityananda in front of a Sri Yantra

Both Rudi and Muktananda were students of, and received diksha (spiritual initiation) from, the great Indian saint Bhagavan Nityananda. Nityananda is thus considered the root guru, or "great-grandfather," of Shambhavananda's lineage. He was a great siddha, or perfected being. Shambhavananda says that Nityananda was such a great being that he will continue to affect people for hundreds of years. He describes Nityananda as having "brought everything to us," and our connection to him as "a living connection." He says Nityananda's grace flows where there is love and an opening in the heart for it.

Once during a visit, Muktananda told Shambhavananda that someday he would have an ashram on a large piece of land in the mountains, where he would give transmission of spiritual energy to thousands of seekers from all over the world. At the time, he just looked at Muktananda with amazement. He couldn't even fathom such a thing. Time proved Muktananda's vision to be true.

Shambhavananda was awarded the title of Rishi Maha Mandaleshwar by Matri Acharya Maha Mandaleshwar Mataji Ma Yoga Shakti Saraswati of Niranjani Akhara of India. The title Maha Mandaleshwar means the Head of a Circle (Mandala) of Swamis. It is a title of great respect given to spiritual masters in the yogic tradition. One who is called Maha Mandaleshwar has been elevated by his peers to the highest level of traditional spiritual guardianship. Niranjani Akhara is the oldest, largest, and most active organization of swamis and sadhus in the world, and Shambhavananda is one of the first Americans in history to be awarded this title.

Shoshoni Yoga Retreat was founded by Sri Shambhavananda as a residential yoga ashram and retreat center located in a spectacular setting in the Rocky Mountains near Boulder, Colorado. Shoshoni is a place of spiritual pilgrimage for people from all over the world and home to a group of dedicated yogis. Shambhavananda has been serving the local community for over thirty years by offering spiritual teachings, places of sanctuary, and training programs in hatha yoga and meditation.

Shambhavananda's teachings are derived from the ancient philosophy of Kashmir Saivism. Swami Muktananda once said that of all the profound yogic doctrines, Kashmir Saivism is the most consistent with his own personal experience. This mystical path has produced many great siddhas, such as Bhagavan Nityananda and Swami Muktananda. It teaches that freedom is as natural to us as the breath; we only have to recognize it. Meditation and a personal relationship with the guru are what allow us to clear away our misunderstandings and awaken to our innate divinity.

Hatha Yoga and Meditation in the Shambhava School

Shambhava hatha yoga is yoga from the heart. It is a classic hatha yoga that brings us back to inner awareness and to the breath. Shambhava hatha yoga is appropriate for beginner, intermediate, and advanced practitioners. It is the perfect preparation for clearer, deeper, more meaningful meditation experiences.

Because meditation is a core practice in the Shambhava School, it colors the way hatha yoga practice is presented. Meditation is a practice that involves turning our attention from the external world, the world we normally experience with our senses, to look inside. It involves deeply letting go of thoughts, fantasies, emotions, and deeper psychic tensions. It involves freeing ourselves from our total absorption in the swirling world around us in order to experience who we are beyond these fluctuations of the mind and senses. What we find inside has many names. In the Shambhava School we call it the Inner Self. Sri Shambhavananda describes the Inner Self as a state of being, an experience of profound happiness and clarity. Classically described as sat-chit-ananda (being,

13

consciousness, and bliss), this state exists within everyone, and meditation is a means of realizing this state. How do we know this state exists inside us and is not found in what we experience outside us? Shambhavananda says that if happiness were to be found in the objects in the world around us, then the more of these objects we have the happier we'd be. He often compares such happiness with the delight we experience when eating an ice cream sundae. We all know we don't get happier the more ice cream sundaes we eat! The delight we feel is not in the ice cream but comes from inside us. It is a reflection of the Self within. By opening up to the happiness of the Self, our perspective on life and everything in it begins to change. The light of the Self begins to radiate into all corners and aspects of our beings.

The Shambhava School approaches yoga and meditation as part of the journey of spiritual growth. "Spiritual" in this context doesn't refer to something other-worldly; it refers to our most fundamental nature, our true Self. There is no higher or better use for one's life than to dedicate it to becoming happier, more conscious, and more alive. Living consciously will inevitably lead to more consciousness in the people and situations around us. Students often ask Shambhavananda whether meditation is a religion. He says that meditation is a process that no religion can own. It is a process of accessing a deeper level of consciousness, which is the source of our energy. This process is a practice we take into the heart of our lives, whatever our circumstances, until the practice actually becomes our life. Shambhava meditation is a sacred journey of Self-realization, a process that ulti-

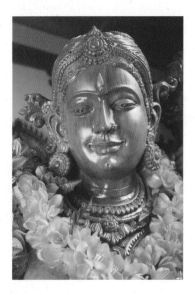

mately leads to the recognition that we and the world around us are one and the same energy. This understanding may dawn slowly, or it may blaze from within that our nature is consciousness itself, the very same consciousness that exists in everyone and everything. The practices of yoga and meditation are what create the opening for real understanding to come.

General Overview of the Subtle Body in Hatha Yoga

According to yogic philosophy, a human being is not just a physical body but a collection of three subtle bodies, which consist of more and more refined energy. These are referred to as the subtle, causal, and supracausal bodies. They correspond to levels of consciousness that we experience every day. The physical body corresponds to the waking state. The subtle body corresponds to dreaming. The causal body relates to deep sleep, and the supercausal body is associated with the deepest state of pure consciousness.

The physical body is a denser, manifest form of energy that is dominated by the world of the senses. The subtle body is the realm of mind, emotions, and prana (vital life force). The causal body holds the deep unconscious storehouse of past impressions that are purified and released through spiritual practice. Hatha yoga asanas begin the process of purification within the subtle body. Through this process, the chakras (spiritual energy centers) begin to open through the natural process of growth. Eventually this leads to the merging of all of our bodies into the highest state of consciousness, known as samadhi.

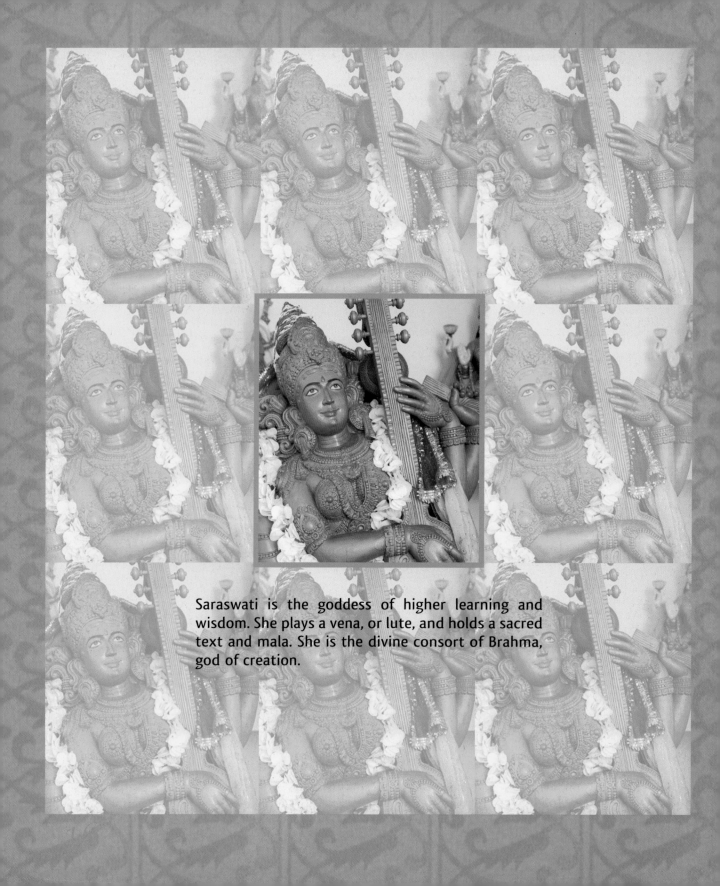

Saraswati is the goddess of higher learning and wisdom. She plays a vena, or lute, and holds a sacred text and mala. She is the divine consort of Brahma, god of creation.

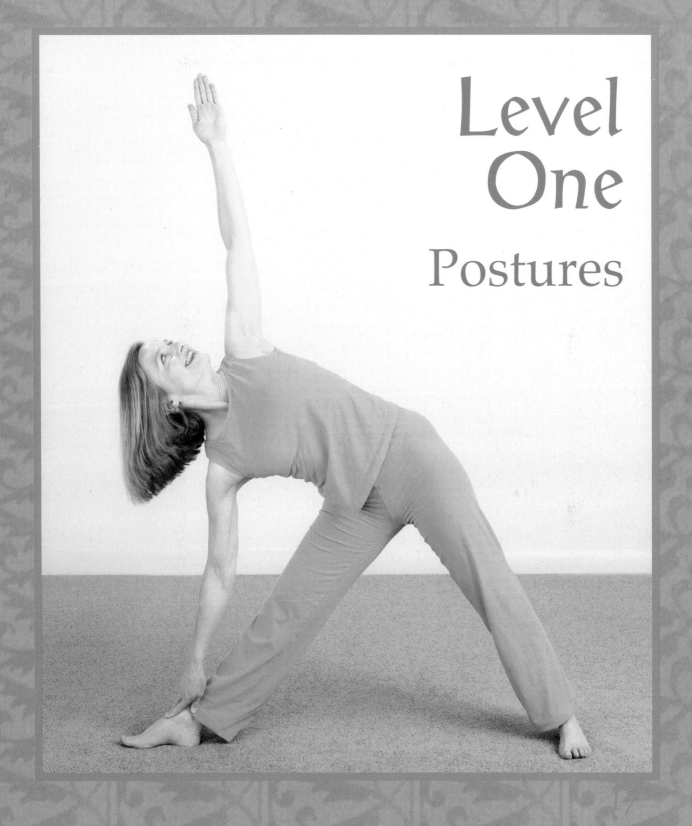

Level One
Postures

Introduction to the Postures

The goal of hatha yoga may be samadhi (state of enlightenment); however, it is the daily journey to that inner state of consciousness that brings about balance. Balance is created by bringing together opposite qualities, such as creating an experience of serenity in a very active person or creating an experience of aliveness and vitality in a very sedentary person. At first, beginners have to learn how to position their bodies and breathe correctly in the poses. Later, experienced practitioners can reach within to develop a deeper awareness in each pose. Working in this way, the practice always feels fresh and new. The pose is an expression of our thoughts, attitudes, intentions, and focus. Because of this, it is expressed in a unique way each time it is practiced. The purpose of aligning the bones and muscles in a specific way in a posture is to allow the underlying tensions to dissolve with the energy and focus of the breath. Because of this, even a brief daily practice will leave you feeling relaxed and renewed.

How Do You Know if Your Practice Is Effective?

You know if your practice is going well if you feel content and happy. Sri Shambhavananda has said that hatha yoga is a spiritual practice if done consciously and with the breath. It is just exercise if done without these things. "I have seen people do the Sun Salutation, and it was so beautiful to watch because there was such surrender and devotion and awareness. Any movement done consciously is yoga."

To bring conscious focus to your practice, simply begin a posture by remembering why you want to practice and what brought you to do yoga. Breathe deeply, noticing the effects of the breath, and become quiet. A natural joy arises from the quiet within, which you can increase with feelings of loving-kindness toward yourself and others. From this center, begin the postures, moving with the breath. Inhale to open and expand while stretching, and exhale to close, twist, or contract in a posture. Maintain the calmness within as you practice each posture for one to two minutes, using either many repetitions or just one. Your awareness and movement will harmonize with the natural pulses of life. As thoughts and emotions arise, just let them go, as a cloud passes in the sky. This is the inner secret of surrender that allows you to simply experience hatha yoga.

While yoga helps open you up to discover the happiness within, the natural joy of life is a chosen lifestyle. Sri Shambhavananda describes it like this: "The reason I stay pretty happy is because my joy does not come from something outside of me; it comes from a place that I have found inside. I look at the moon in the morning when I get up, and it makes me happy. Peacefulness comes from understanding the nature of the world. It is the way you live life and your connectedness that brings you happiness."

If you cultivate a regular hatha yoga practice with the intention of becoming more happy, healthy, and balanced, then you will always look forward to doing it. You will always find the time, the place, and a way to do your practice. It will be a highlight of your day.

Build Your Own Practice

Hatha yoga practice can be customized to help each individual find his or her optimal balance. First, determine how to bring balance to your own practice by noting your current lifestyle, physical condition, and temperament. Make a list of the opposite qualities, including a list of postures that help you to feel these qualities. For example: Current lifestyle, on the go. Opposite quality to create balance: Relaxation with restorative yoga.

Second, create your own routine using the simple formula below. Include some poses you like, as well as some poses that you feel neutral about and others that you like to avoid. Be sure to include the postures that you wrote down to bring balancing qualities to your practice. Add a short warm-up, such as the Shambhava Leg and Hip Stretches (pages 202-205), and a brief cool down, such as an easy reclined twist (such as Supine Cross-Legged Twist, page 205) and Wind Reliever (page 48). Then remain in the resting pose, Savasana (page 206), for three minutes to relax.

Create a Thirty-Minute Routine

	POSTURE FAMILY	EXAMPLES
1	dynamic series	Sun Salutation (pages 76-79), or Staff of Brahma (pages 74-75)
2 to 3	standing poses	Warrior 2 (page 28), Triangle (page 30)
1	standing balance pose	Tree (page 32) or Half Moon (page 36)
1 to 2	forward bending poses	Single Leg Forward Bend (page 43), Double Leg Forward Bend (page 42)
1	twisting pose	Half Spinal Twist (page 52) or Hip Spiral (page 53)
1 to 2	backward bending poses	Simple Fish (page 65), Bridge Pose (page 64)
1 to 2	inverted poses	Shoulderstand (page 70), Plow (page 71)
1	hand balance	Handstand (page 144) or Crane with Leg Extended (page 185)
	cool down	
	relaxation	

Relaxation

Develop your own practice by going through each chapter, trying the poses (as long as you are comfortable with them), the breathing exercises, the meditation practices, and the Home Practice Sequences. Choose your favorites. Then customize a yoga routine, and add a breathing exercise and a meditation practice. It can be as easy, relaxing, or as challenging as you want.

Explanation of Terms Used in the Posture Chapters

After most posture descriptions is a list of brief reminders and helpful information about the pose. These include:

GAZE   WARM-UPS   COUNTERPOSES   EASY VARIATIONS   BENEFITS   BREATHING

GAZE: Where to set your eyes or focus as you practice.

WARM-UPS: Suggested postures or easy stretches that help you prepare for the pose.

COUNTERPOSES: Suggested postures or easy stretches that help your muscles regain balance after you practice the pose.

EASY VARIATIONS: Alternatives or modifications to help you achieve the pose.

BENEFITS: The beneficial effects of the pose.

BREATHING: A helpful review of the breathing suggested for the pose.

Explanation of General Terms Used throughout the Posture Chapters

ACTIVATE: To tighten the muscles and prepare your body to move.

BEND: To move your body at the joint.

CAT-COW: Begin in Table Pose (on hands and knees) and inhale. Arch to look up. Exhale, rounding the back to look down.

CRESCENT STRETCH: Stand in Mountain Pose (page 26). Inhale while reaching the arms forward and up overhead. Arch back while gently tightening the buttocks.

EASY SITTING POSE: Sit upright with your legs folded comfortably on the floor.

EASY SIT-UPS: Any easy abdominal curl such as: Begin on your back and interlace your fingers behind the head. Bend your knees and place the feet flat on the floor. Tighten the abdominal muscles and exhale while curling up, elbows toward the knees. Inhale while relaxing the head back down to the floor.

Half Lotus: Position one ankle at the hip crease of the opposite leg.

Hip Cradle: Hip stretch that is generally done in the sitting position. Hold one lower leg between your elbows and gently rock from side to side to increase hip flexibility.

Lunges: While standing, separate your feet about three feet apart and bend one knee over the ankle to create a stretch in your leg and hips.

Prayer Position: Bring both hands to the heart with palms together.

Reclined Hip Twist: Supine cross-legged twist.

Sit Bones: The right and left ischial tuberosities, which are the boney protuberances at the base of the hip. These are known as the "sit bones" because they support the pelvis when we sit down.

Sitting Child's Pose: Sit upright and hug both knees to the chest. Relax the head to rest on the knees.

Square the Hips: To position your hips in the same forward alignment as your shoulders. This position makes many postures easier to perform.

Square the Hips Forward: To position your hips in the same forward direction as your shoulders.

STAFF POSE: Sit upright with both of your legs extended and the ankles together. Place the hands palms down on each side of the hips. The body is alert and active, but not moving.

STANDING HIP STRETCHES: Stand and draw the right knee up and catch your hands around the knee. Stretch the hip by hugging the knee in toward the shoulder. Exhale and release the right foot, lowering it back down to the floor.

STANDING STRADDLE: While standing, separate your feet about three feet apart with your feet parallel.

TABLE POSE: Begin on all fours, placing the hands below the shoulders and the hips above the knees.

T-POSITION: Extend the arms perpendicular to the body, creating the shape of the letter T.

PLANE: The alignment of the legs, hips, back, shoulders, neck, and head in a single plane, as though you were leaning against Plexiglas.

Chapter One

Beginning Postures

"Practice being happy." – Faith Stone

These are the foundational postures for beginning hatha yoga practitioners. Practicing these postures will provide strength and flexibility. Learn each by practicing until it becomes easy to breathe in the posture, and you can comfortably hold it for about six breaths. Move with the breath in each posture, generally inhaling for expanding movements and exhaling for contracting movements. Use the Abdominal Breathing and Ujjayi Breath (page 82) techniques while practicing these postures. When you are comfortable with this posture set and the Hatha Yoga Practice Sequences listed on pages 84 and 85, continue to the Level Two Postures.

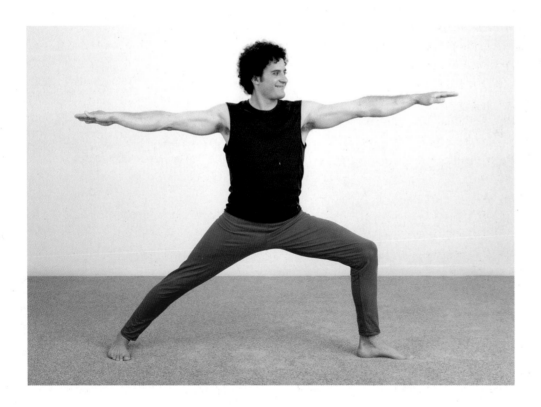

MOUNTAIN

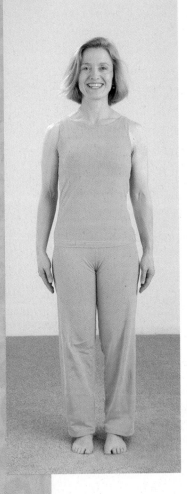

1. Begin standing at the front end of the yoga mat. Position your feet hip distance apart. Imagine a line from your small toe to the heel of both feet and bring your feet parallel to each other.

2. Vertically align your ankles, knees, hip joints, shoulder joints, and ears. Gently lift up through the top of your head.

3. Gently rotate your thighs inward. Tuck in your pelvis slightly to help lengthen your spine.

4. Activate both the front and back of your torso. Lift through your sternum to open your chest area. Gently expand through the back of your ribs to balance your chest expansion. A relaxed, deep breath will lift your spine and lightly expand the front and back of your torso.

5. Roll your shoulders toward your spine to relax your shoulder blades. Bring your hands to the sides of your body. Gently stretch through your fingers.

6. Remain in the pose, breathing steadily. Make slight adjustments as needed to maintain a quiet mind and quiet pose.

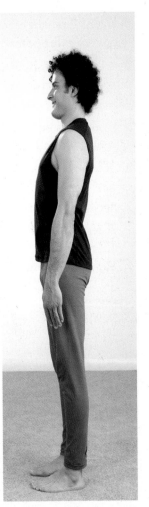

Gaze:	Center of the forehead.
Warm-ups:	Twisting Bear (page 197).
Counterpose:	Standing Forward Bend (page 37).
Easy variation:	Sit in a chair and quiet your mind.
Benefits:	Increases inner awareness and balance.
Breathing:	Steady.

WARRIOR I

1. Begin in Mountain (page 26) at the front end of the yoga mat. Inhale and lengthen your spine. Exhale and bring your right foot back about three feet. Angle your toes forward so your foot is comfortable. Align your front toes and heel with the arch of the back foot.

2. Square your hips forward. Tuck in your pelvis slightly to lengthen your spine.

3. Inhale and raise your arms over your shoulders, aligning them with your ears. Rotate your palms toward each other.

4. Exhale and lunge, bringing your front knee over your ankle for support.

5. Press down through your back foot. Keep your hips squared forward. Continue to breathe steadily.

6. Inhale and straighten your front leg to come out of the pose. Exhale and simultaneously release your hands, lowering them down to your sides and stepping forward into Mountain (page 26).

7. Repeat on your left side.

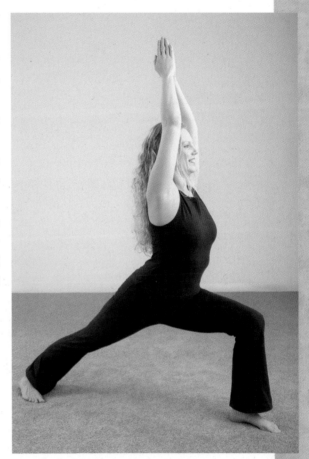

Gaze:	Center of the forehead.
Warm-ups:	Lunges (page 22).
Counterpose:	Standing Forward Bend (page 37).
Easy variation:	Lift your back heel.
Benefits:	Stretches and strengthens the hip, back, and shoulders.
Breathing:	Inhale to lengthen your spine. Exhale, step your foot back. Inhale, raise your arms. Exhale, lunge with your front knee over your ankle. Inhale, straighten your front leg. Exhale, lower your arms and step forward.

WARRIOR II

1. Stand in Mountain (page 26) in the center of the yoga mat. Separate your feet in a wide straddle, about one leg's length apart. Begin on the right. Rotate your right foot out ninety degrees and your left foot in thirty degrees. Inhale and draw your arms up parallel to the floor. Square your hips forward and gently tuck in your pelvis.

2. Exhale and bend your front knee over your ankle, keeping your arms parallel to the floor.

3. Stay in the pose for four to six breaths, breathing steadily, with your front thigh parallel to the floor. Work to open the hips by keeping your front knee over the ankle and your back hip squared forward.

4. Inhale and lift out of the pose to the Standing Straddle Forward Bend (page 38). Rotate your feet back.

5. Exhale and step into Mountain (page 26). Repeat on your left side.

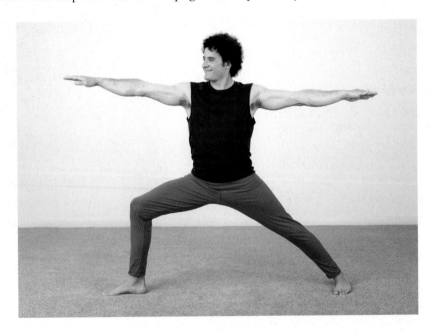

Gaze:	Center of the forehead.
Warm-ups:	Lunges (page 22), Standing Straddle Forward Bend (page 38).
Counterposes:	Single Leg Forward Bend (page 43), Standing Forward Bend (page 37).
Easy variation:	Shorten your stance; place your hands on your hips.
Benefits:	Stretches and strengthens the hip, back, and shoulders.
Breathing:	Inhale, draw your arms up and lengthen your spine. Exhale, lunge with your front knee over your ankle. Inhale, straighten your front leg. Exhale, lower your arms and step forward.

LATERAL ANGLE

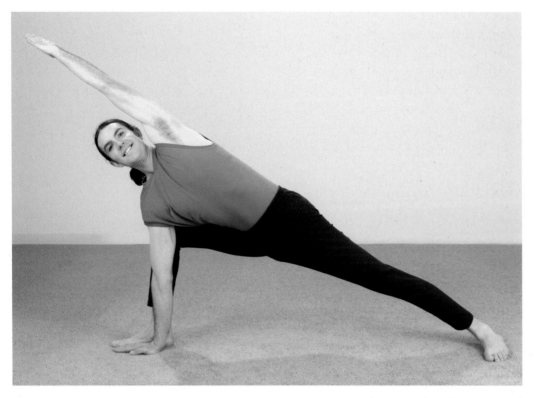

1. Begin in Mountain (page 26) in the center of the yoga mat. Separate your feet in a wide straddle. Rotate your right foot out ninety degrees and your left foot in thirty degrees. Inhale and draw your arms up parallel to the floor.

2. Exhale and bend your front knee over your ankle, and lower your right hand to the floor in front of your right foot. Inhale and extend your left arm up over your left ear, palm down.

3. Stay in the pose with your front thigh parallel to the floor, working to open your left hip and maintain one plane from your left ankle to your left hand.

4. Inhale and lift out of the pose to the Standing Straddle (page 23). Exhale and step into Mountain (page 26). Repeat on the other side.

Gaze:	Look up.
Warm-ups:	Warrior II (page 28), Standing Forward Bend (page 37), Standing Head to Knee with Belt (page 41).
Counterposes:	Standing Forward Bend (page 37), Standing Straddle Forward Bend (page 38).
Easy variation:	Lower your forearm onto your thigh instead of reaching for the floor.
Benefits:	Increases strength and flexibility for hips, back, legs, and shoulders.
Breathing:	Exhale into the pose. Inhale out of the pose.

TRIANGLE

1. Begin in Mountain (page 26) in the center of the yoga mat. Separate your feet in a wide straddle. Begin on the right side. Rotate your right foot out ninety degrees and your left foot in thirty degrees. Inhale and draw your arms up parallel to the floor.

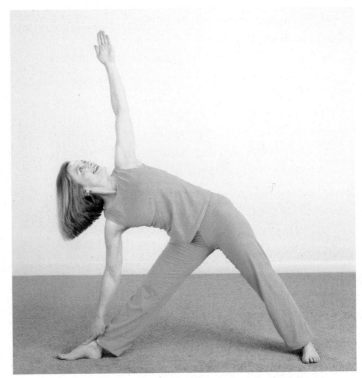

2. Exhale and bend laterally. Push your left hip back and bend to the right, keeping the body in one plane. Place your right hand on your lower leg, ankle, or the floor (inside your foot). Reach your left hand straight up, palm rotated forward. Keep your emphasis on the hip stretch.

3. Remain in the pose for four to six breaths, breathing steadily. Work to open your hip and lengthen your spine.

4. Inhale and lift your shoulders to come out of the pose. Rotate your feet forward.

5. Exhale and step back into Mountain (page 26). Repeat on the other side.

Gaze:	Upper hand.
Warm-ups:	Lunges (page 22), Standing Straddle Forward Bend (page 38), Warrior II (page 28).
Counterposes:	Standing Forward Bend (page 37), Standing Straddle Forward Bend (page 38).
Easy variation:	Shorten your stance; place your hands on your hips.
Benefits:	Stretches and strengthens the hip, back, and shoulders.
Breathing:	Inhale, draw your arms up and lengthen your spine. Exhale, bend to the side. Inhale, draw your shoulders up. Exhale, lower your arms and bring your feet together.

REVOLVED TRIANGLE

1. Begin in Mountain (page 26) at the front end of the yoga mat. Inhale and lengthen your spine. Exhale and step your right foot back about three feet. Angle your toes forward so your foot is comfortable. Align your front toes and heel with the arch of your back foot.

2. Square your hips forward. Tuck in your pelvis slightly to lengthen your spine.

3. Inhale and raise your arms parallel to the floor.

4. Exhale and rotate your left hand first to your right knee. Place your right hand on your right hip.

5. Slowly ease into the full pose by rotating your spine a little more and hinging forward a little more.

6. Once in the full pose, place your left hand on the floor to the outside of your right foot. Inhale and raise your right arm straight up, fingers pointing upward. Rotate your head to gaze upward.

7. Exhale and release your right arm, lowering it down to the floor and begin coming out of the pose. Steady yourself.

8. Inhale and raise your shoulders up. Exhale and release your arms to your sides while stepping into Mountain (page 26). Repeat on the other side.

Gaze:	Upper hand.
Warm-ups:	Lunges (page 22), Standing Straddle Forward Bend (page 38), Warrior II (page 28), Triangle (page 30).
Counterposes:	Standing Forward Bend (page 37), Standing Straddle Forward Bend (page 38).
Easy variation:	Shorten the stance; place your right hand on your right hip and your left hand on your right knee.
Benefits:	Stretches and strengthens the hip, back, and shoulders.
Breathing:	Inhale, draw your arms up and lengthen your spine. Exhale, rotate and bend into the pose. Inhale, draw your top arm up. Exhale, lower your top arm. Inhale, draw your shoulder up. Exhale, lower your arms and bring your feet together.

TREE

1. Begin standing. Tuck in your pelvis, activate your legs, and shift your weight onto your right foot.
2. Raise your left foot and lightly rest it at your right knee.
3. Bring your hands together in front of your heart or inhale and extend them over your shoulders, palms rotated toward each other.
4. With steady breathing, allow your mind to become still.
5. Exhale and release from the pose. Repeat on the other side.

Variation 1

1. Begin in Mountain (page 26) at the front end of the yoga mat. Tuck in your pelvis, activate your legs, and shift your weight onto your right foot.
2. Raise your left foot and press it against your right thigh with your toes pointing down.
3. Bring your hands together in front of your heart, or inhale and extend your hands over your shoulders with your palms rotated toward each other.
4. With steady breathing, allow your mind to become still.
5. Exhale and release from the pose. Repeat on the other side.

Variation 2

1. Begin in Mountain (page 26) at the front end of the yoga mat. Tuck in your pelvis, activate your legs, and shift your weight onto your right foot.
2. Raise your left foot into Half Lotus (page 89) and rest it on the top of your right thigh.
3. Bring your hands together in front of your heart, or inhale and extend your hands over your shoulders with your palms rotated toward each other.
4. With steady breathing, allow your mind to become still.
5. Exhale and release from the pose. Repeat on the other side.

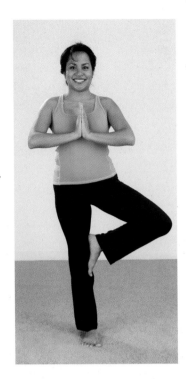

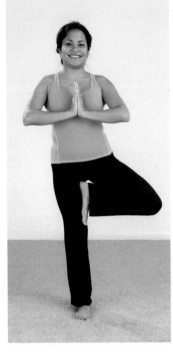

Variation 1

Variation 2

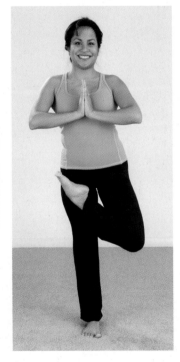

Gaze:	Center of the forehead.
Warm-ups:	Twisting Bear (page 197), Warrior II (page 28), Triangle (page 30).
Counterpose:	Standing Forward Bend (page 37).
Easy variation:	Place your elevated foot at the inside of your opposite ankle.
Benefits:	Increases inner awareness and balance; hip stretch.
Breathing:	Steady.

WARRIOR III

1. Begin in Mountain (page 26) at the front end of the yoga mat. Shift your weight onto your right side and extend your left foot back one foot. Activate your legs and buttocks. Square your hips forward.

2. Inhale and stretch your arms over your shoulders, with your palms rotated toward each other. Straighten your right leg.

3. Exhale and bend forward, bringing your arms, back, and left leg parallel to the floor. Breathe steadily.

4. Inhale, lift your shoulders, and lower your left leg.

5. Exhale and release your arms and legs into Mountain (page 26). Repeat on the other side.

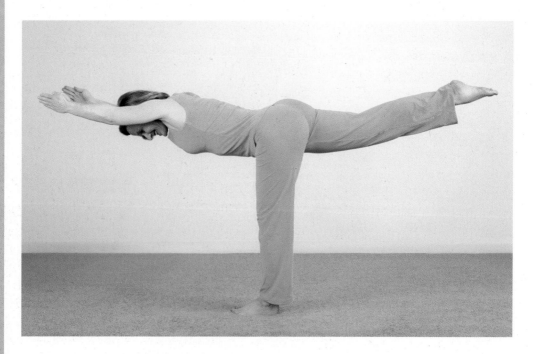

Gaze:	Center of the forehead.
Warm-ups:	Lunges (page 22), Warrior I (page 27).
Counterposes:	Standing Forward Bend (page 37), Twisting Bear (page 197).
Easy variation:	Reach forward, resting your hands on a chair for balance.
Benefits:	Stretches and strengthens the legs, hip, back, and shoulders.
Breathing:	Inhale, draw your arms up and lengthen your spine. Exhale, bend forward into the balance. Inhale, raise your arms. Exhale, lower your arms and step forward.

DANCER

1. Begin in Mountain (page 26) at the front end of the yoga mat. Shift your weight onto your right side and reach back for your left foot with your left arm. Activate your right leg and left buttock. Square your hips forward.

2. Inhale, stretch your right arm over your shoulder with your palm rotated toward your ear, while lifting your left thigh parallel to the floor.

3. Exhale and release from the pose, bringing your arms and legs down into Mountain (page 26). Repeat on the other side.

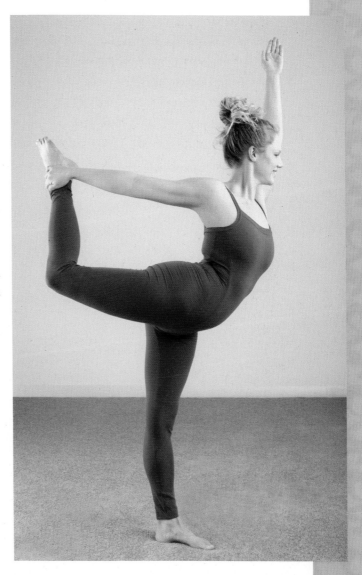

Gaze:	Center of the forehead.
Warm-ups:	Lunges (page 22), Quad Stretch at Wall (page 198), Sun Salutations (pages 76-79).
Counterposes:	Standing Forward Bend (page 37), Twisting Bear (page 197).
Easy variation:	Use a yoga strap looped around your foot to raise your back leg.
Benefits:	Stretches and strengthens the hip, back, and shoulders.
Breathing:	Inhale to lengthen your spine and draw your back leg up. Exhale, release your foot back down.

HALF MOON

1. Begin in Mountain (page 26) in the center of the yoga mat. Separate your feet in a wide straddle. Begin on the right. Rotate your right foot out ninety degrees and your left foot in thirty degrees. Inhale and draw your arms up parallel to the floor.

2. Exhale and bend your right knee over your right ankle, and lower your right hand to the floor, reaching in front of your right foot.

3. Inhale, extend and lift your left leg up, pressing up through your ankle bone. Straighten your right leg. Draw your left arm straight up, palm rotated forward.

4. Stay in the pose for four to six breaths, working to open the left hip and maintain one plane. Steady breathing will help you stay balanced.

5. Exhale and lower your left arm and leg into a Lunge (page 22).

6. Inhale and lift out of the pose to the Standing Straddle (page 23). Exhale and step into Mountain (page 26). Repeat on the other side.

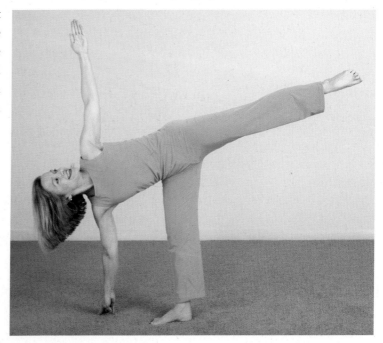

Gaze:	Top hand.
Warm-ups:	Lunges (page 22), Warrior II (page 28), Triangle (page 30), Sun Salutations (pages 76-79).
Counterposes:	Standing Forward Bend (page 37), Downward Facing Dog (page 73).
Easy variation:	Resting Side Pose (page 114).
Benefits:	Stretches and strengthens the hip, back, and shoulders; massages the sacral nerve plexus.
Breathing:	Inhale to lengthen your spine and draw your arms up. Exhale, reach your front hand to the floor. Inhale, draw your back leg and top arm up. Exhale, release your top arm and leg. Inhale, raise your shoulders. Exhale, lower your arms and bring your feet together.

STANDING FORWARD BEND

1. Begin in Mountain (page 26) at the front end of the yoga mat. Position your feet parallel to each other, hip distance apart.

2. Vertically align your ankles, knees, hip joints, shoulder joints, and ears. Gently lift up through the top of your head.

3. Gently rotate your thighs inward. Tuck in your pelvis slightly to help lengthen your spine.

4. Inhale and raise your arms above your shoulders, with your palms rotated toward each other.

5. Exhale, bend forward, and place your hands on your lower legs, ankles, or heels. Keep your head, neck, and spine aligned. Tighten your abdominal muscles for support.

6. Inhale, release from the pose, and draw your shoulders back up. Raise your arms either straight up, aligned with your ears, or sweep them out to the sides and overhead.

7. Exhale and lower your arms to your sides.

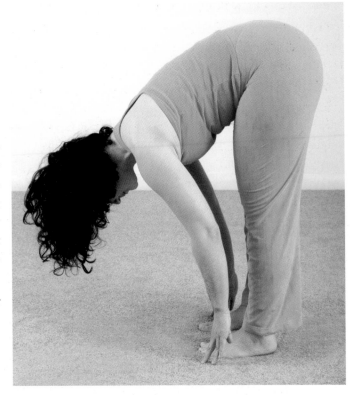

Gaze:	Center of the forehead.
Warm-ups:	Lunges (page 22), Warrior I (page 27), Sun Salutations (pages 76-79).
Counterpose:	Twisting Bear (page 197).
Easy variation:	Bend the knees.
Benefits:	Stretches the hamstring muscles, hip, back, and shoulders.
Breathing:	Inhale, draw your arms up and lengthen your spine. Exhale, bend forward. Inhale, raise your arms and shoulders. Exhale, lower your arms to your sides.

STANDING STRADDLE FORWARD BEND

1. Begin in Mountain (page 26) in the center of the yoga mat. Position your feet parallel to each other, one leg's distance apart.

2. Gently rotate the thighs inward. Tuck in your pelvis slightly to help lengthen your spine.

3. Inhale and raise your arms above your shoulders, with your palms rotated toward each other.

4. Exhale, bend forward, and lower your hands first to the floor underneath your shoulders. Lower further, as flexibility allows, sliding your hands back, palms down, to align your fingertips with your toes. Lower your head to the floor, placing it between both hands. Keep your head, neck, and spine aligned. Tighten your abdominal muscles for support.

5. Inhale, release from the pose, and draw your shoulders back up. Raise your arms either straight up, aligned with your ears, or sweep them out to your sides and overhead.

6. Exhale and lower your arms to your sides. Step into Mountain (page 26).

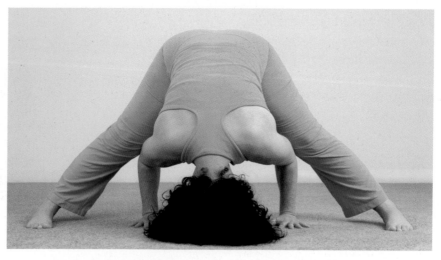

Gaze:	Center of the forehead.
Warm-ups:	Lunges (page 22), Warrior II (page 28), Triangle (page 30).
Counterpose:	Crescent Stretch (page 21).
Easy variation:	Bend your knees; place your hands on your knees.
Benefits:	Stretches the hamstring muscles, hip, back, and shoulders.
Breathing:	Inhale, draw your arms up and lengthen your spine. Exhale, bend forward. Inhale, raise your arms and shoulders. Exhale, lower your arms to your sides.

STANDING HEAD TO KNEE

1. Begin in Mountain (page 26) at the end of the yoga mat. Inhale and lengthen your spine. Exhale and step your right foot back about three feet. Angle your toes forward so your foot is comfortable. Align your toes and heel with the arch of your back foot.

2. Square your hips forward. (The proper hip placement will prevent rotation and rounding of the spine.) Tuck in your pelvis slightly to lengthen your spine.

3. Interlace your hands at the base of your spine. Inhale and lift through your chest in a slight initial arch to extend your spine.

4. Exhale and bend forward. Raise your arms over your shoulders, lowering your chin below your knee. Keep your head, neck, and spine aligned.

5. Press down through your back foot. Keep your hips squared. Continue to breathe steadily.

6. Inhale and lift your shoulders to come out of the pose. Exhale and simultaneously release your hands down to your sides while stepping forward into Mountain (page 26).

7. Repeat on your left side.

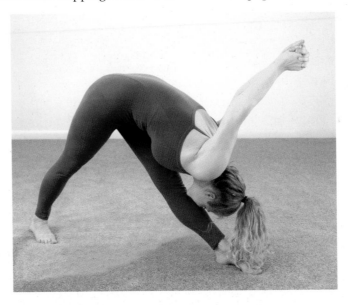

Gaze:	Center of the forehead.
Warm-ups:	Warrior I (page 27), Sun Salutations (pages 76-79).
Counterposes:	Twisting Bear (page 197), Catcher's Stretch (page 197).
Easy variation:	Shorten the stance; use a yoga belt.
Benefits:	Stretches the hamstring muscles, hip, back, and shoulders.
Breathing:	Inhale, draw your arms up and lift your chest. Exhale, bend forward. Inhale, raise your arms and shoulders. Exhale, lower your arms to your sides and bring your feet together.

STANDING HEAD TO KNEE

WITH REVERSE NAMASTE

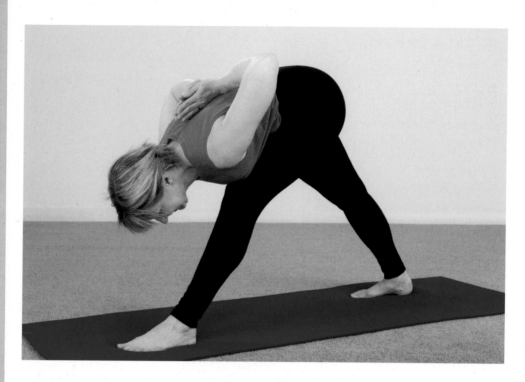

1. Begin in Mountain (page 26) at the end of the yoga mat. Inhale and lengthen your spine. Exhale and step your right foot back about three feet. Angle your toes forward so your foot is comfortable. Align your front toes and heel with the arch of your back foot.

2. Square your hips forward. (The proper hip placement will prevent rotation and rounding in of the spine.) Tuck in your pelvis slightly to lengthen your spine.

3. Bring your hands into prayer position between your shoulder blades. Inhale and lift through your chest in a slight initial arch to extend your spine.

4. Exhale and bend forward. Raise your arms over your shoulders, lowering your chin below your knee. Keep your head, neck, and spine aligned.

5. Press down through your back foot. Keep your hips squared. Continue to breathe steadily.

6. Inhale and lift your shoulders to come out of the pose. Exhale and simultaneously release your hands down to your sides while stepping forward into Mountain (page 26).

7. Repeat on your left side.

STANDING HEAD TO KNEE
WITH BELT

1. Begin in Mountain (page 26) at the end of the yoga mat. Inhale and lengthen your spine. Exhale and step your right foot back about two feet. Angle your toes forward so your foot is comfortable. Align your front toes and heel with your back arch.

2. Square your hips forward. (The proper hip placement will prevent rotation and rounding in of the spine.) Tuck in your pelvis slightly to lengthen your spine.

3. Catch hold of a yoga belt behind your back for an easier shoulder stretch. Inhale and draw the belt up behind your back. Exhale and bend into Standing Head to Knee (page 39).

4. Lower your chin below your knee. Keep your head, neck, and spine aligned.

5. Press down through your back foot. Keep your hips squared. Continue to breathe steadily.

6. Inhale and lift your shoulders to come out of the pose. Exhale and simultaneously release your hands down to your sides while stepping forward into Mountain (page 26).

7. Repeat on your left side.

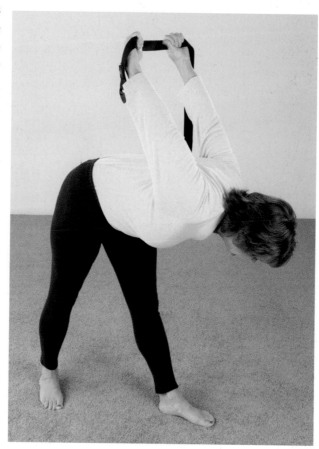

DOUBLE LEG FORWARD BEND

1. Begin sitting on the yoga mat with both legs extended forward. Keep your ankles and toes together. Slightly rotate your thighs inward to activate your inner leg muscles.

2. Inhale and draw your arms up over your shoulders, with your palms rotated toward each other.

3. Exhale and bend forward, keeping your head, neck, and spine in line. Release your hands and place them on either your lower legs, ankles, or heels.

4. For a deeper stretch, grasp your heels and lower your elbows to the floor. Bring your forearms alongside your lower legs. Position your chin below your knees and forehead on your lower leg. Breathe steadily.

5. Inhale, lift your arms parallel to your ears, and bring your shoulders upright.

6. Exhale and lower your arms to your sides.

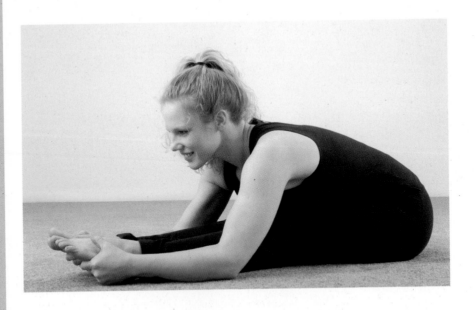

Gaze:	Center of the forehead.
Warm-ups:	Warrior I (page 27), Standing Head to Knee (page 39), Standing Forward Bend (page 37).
Counterposes:	Sitting Hip Rolls (page 199), Half Spinal Twist (page 52).
Easy variation:	Bend your knees; use a yoga belt.
Benefits:	Stretches the hamstring muscles; invigorating for the hip, back, and shoulders.
Breathing:	Inhale, draw your arms up. Exhale, bend forward. Inhale, raise your arms and shoulders. Exhale, lower your arms to your sides.

SINGLE LEG FORWARD BEND

1. Begin sitting on the yoga mat with your right leg extended. Activate your right leg.

2. Inhale and draw your arms up over your shoulders, with your palms rotated in toward each other.

3. Exhale and bend forward, keeping your head, neck, and spine in line. Release your hands and place them on either your lower leg, ankle, or heel.

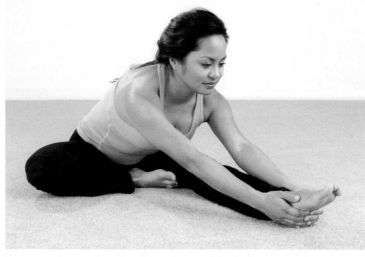

4. For a deeper stretch, grasp your heel and lower your elbows to the floor beside your knee. Bring your forearms alongside your lower leg. Position your chin below your knee, placing your forehead on your lower leg. Breathe steadily.

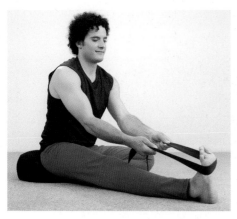

5. Inhale, lift your arms parallel to your ears, and bring your shoulders upright.

6. Exhale and lower your arms down to your sides. Repeat on the other side.

SINGLE LEG FORWARD BEND WITH BELT

1. Practice the Single Leg Forward Bend (above) and loop a yoga belt over your extended foot.

2. Keep your arms straight. Lift through your chest to keep your head, neck, and spine in one plane.

Gaze:	Center of the forehead.
Warm-ups:	Staff of Brahma (page 74), Standing Straddle Forward Bend (page 38).
Counterposes:	Sitting Hip Rolls (page 199), Half Spinal Twist (page 52), Reverse Plank (page 165).
Easy variation:	Bend your knee; use a yoga belt.
Benefits:	Stretches the hamstring muscles; invigorating for the hip, back, and shoulders.
Breathing:	Inhale, draw your arms up. Exhale, bend forward. Inhale, raise your arms and shoulders. Exhale, lower your arms to your sides.

REVOLVED HEAD TO KNEE (EASY)

1. Begin sitting in the center of the yoga mat with your legs in a wide straddle. Fold your left foot in to rest against your inner right thigh. Activate your legs.

2. Inhale and extend your left arm up over your shoulder, with your palm facing down. Exhale and side bend to the right, going as far as comfort allows.

3. Lower your right forearm to the floor along the inside of your right leg, with your palm facing either up or toward the floor.

4. Inhale and extend through your spine. Exhale, lowering a bit further into the pose. Gently rotate through your ribs to lift your heart.

5. Inhale and raise your shoulders to release from the stretch. Exhale and release your legs back into the Easy Sitting Pose (page 21). Repeat on the other side.

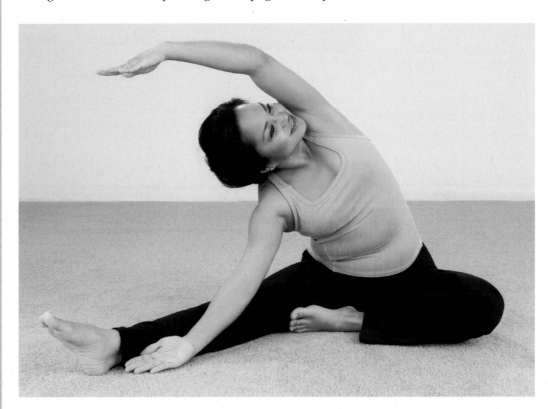

REVOLVED HEAD TO KNEE

1. Begin sitting in the center of the yoga mat with your legs in a wide straddle. Fold your left foot in to rest against your inner right thigh. Activate your legs.

2. Inhale and extend your left arm up over your shoulder, with your palm facing down. Exhale and side bend to the right.

3. Lower your right elbow to the floor along the inside of your right leg, grasping your right big toe.

4. Inhale and extend through your spine. Exhale and lower further into the pose. Grasp your right toe with your left hand. Gently rotate through your ribs to lift your sternum.

5. Exhale and release your hands on your foot and roll forward through your ribs. Inhale and raise your shoulders. Exhale and release your legs back into the Easy Sitting Pose (page 21). Repeat on the other side.

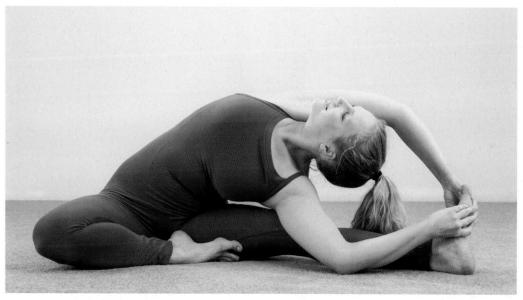

Gaze: Center of the forehead.

Warm-ups: Sun Salutations (pages 76-79), Triangle (page 30), Revolved Triangle (page 31), Lateral Angle Pose (page 29).

Counterposes: Sitting Straddle Forward Bend (page 46), Sitting Hip Rolls (page 199), Wind Reliever (page 48).

Easy variation: Bend the extended leg; side bend comfortably.

Benefits: Stretches the hamstring muscles and hips; strong shoulder, back, and rib stretch.

Breathing: Inhale, lengthen your spine. Exhale, twist toward the folded knee. Inhale, raise your free arm. Exhale, side bend. Inhale, release up from the posture. Exhale, lower your arms to your sides.

SITTING STRADDLE FORWARD BEND

1. Begin sitting in the center of the yoga mat with your legs in a wide straddle. Position your knees and toes up. Draw your sit bones back. Activate your legs.

2. Inhale, lift through your chest and raise your arms over your shoulders.

3. Exhale and bend forward, keeping your head, neck, and spine aligned. Breathe into any areas that feel tight in order to release further into the pose.

4. Inhale and release from the pose, drawing your shoulders up. Exhale and relax your legs into the Easy Sitting Pose (page 21).

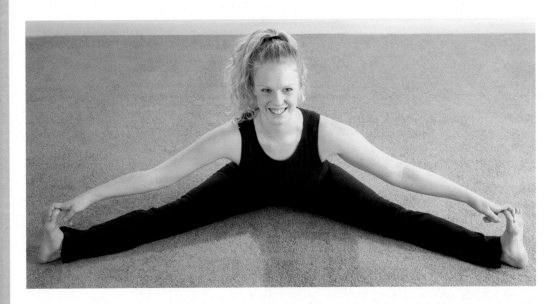

Variation

1. Begin sitting in the center of the yoga mat with your legs in a wide straddle. Position your knees and toes up. Draw your sit bones back. Relax your legs by lifting your knees slightly.

2. Inhale, lift through the chest and raise your arms over your shoulders.

3. Exhale and bend forward, relaxing your back. If needed, place a pillow underneath your sternum for support. Breathe into any tight areas in order to relax further into the pose.

4. Inhale and release from the pose, drawing your shoulders up. Exhale and relax your legs into the Easy Sitting Pose (page 21).

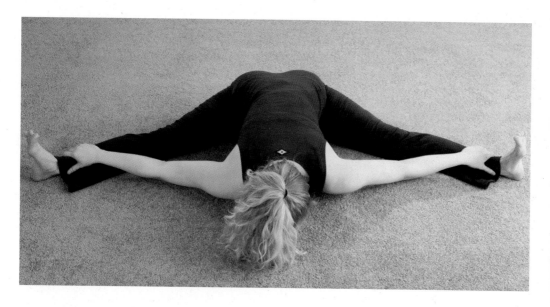

Gaze: Center of the forehead.
Warm-ups: Warrior II (page 28), Catcher's Stretch (page 197), Standing Straddle Forward Bend (page 38).
Counterposes: Sitting Hip Rolls (page 199), Single Leg Forward Bend (page 43), Bridge Pose (page 64).
Easy variation: Bend the knees.
Benefits: Stretches the hamstring and adductor muscles; invigorating for the hip, back, and shoulders.
Breathing: Inhale, draw your arms up. Exhale, bend forward. Inhale, raise your arms and shoulders. Exhale, lower your arms to your sides.

WIND RELIEVER

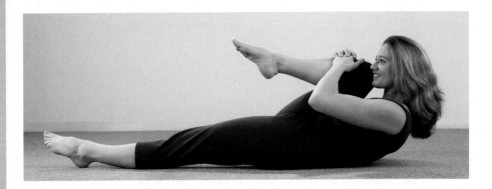

1. Begin by lying on your back, stretched out across the yoga mat. Bend your right leg and catch your hands around your right knee. Inhale and draw the knee toward your shoulder.

2. Exhale and curl up, bringing your right cheek toward your bent knee.

3. Inhale and relax your back to the floor.

4. Exhale and release your knee. Repeat on your left side.

DOUBLE LEG WIND RELIEVER

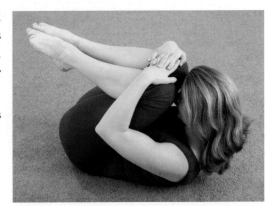

1. Begin by lying on your back, stretched out across the yoga mat. Bend both legs and catch your hands around your knees. Inhale and draw your knees toward your shoulders.

2. Exhale and curl up, bringing your cheeks toward your knees.

3. Inhale and relax your back to the floor.

4. Exhale and release your legs to the floor.

Gaze:	Center of the forehead.
Warm-ups:	Butterfly (page 199), Sitting Hip Rolls (page 199).
Counterposes:	Reclined Hip Rolls (page 54), Double Leg Wind Reliever (page 48).
Easy variation:	Bend the extended leg and place your foot flat on the floor.
Benefits:	Gently stretches the hip, back, and shoulders.
Breathing:	Inhale, draw your knee above your chest. Exhale, curl forward. Inhale, recline. Exhale, relax the pressure on the elevated knee.

CROSSBAR

1. Begin in an upright kneeling position. Shift your weight onto your right knee and extend your left leg to the side. Align your left leg and right knee with the edge of the yoga mat.

2. Inhale and draw your arms up parallel to the floor. Lengthen your spine, square your hips, and tuck in your pelvis.

3. Exhale and bend to the left. Lower your left hand to your lower left leg.

4. Inhale and reach your right hand up beside your ear, with the palm forward. Exhale and stretch further into the pose.

5. Inhale and release from the pose, raising your shoulders. Exhale and release your hands and left leg. Repeat on the other side.

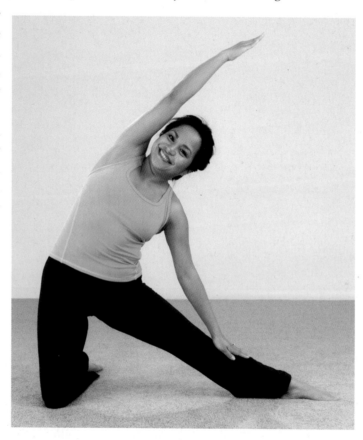

Gaze:	Rotate the head to gaze up. If this is uncomfortable, rotate the head to look down or keep it at center.
Warm-ups:	Warrior II (page 28), Triangle (page 30), Lateral Angle Pose (page 29).
Counterposes:	Devotional Pose (page 207), Rabbit (page 109), Sitting Straddle Forward Bend (page 46).
Easy variation:	Bend the knee on your extended leg.
Benefits:	Stretches the legs, hips, back, and shoulders.
Breathing:	Inhale, draw your arms up parallel to the floor. Exhale, bend to the side. Inhale, raise your arms and shoulders to center. Exhale, lower your arms to your sides.

49

HALF BOAT

1. Begin by resting on your back on the yoga mat with both legs extended forward. Activate your legs. Place your feet together.

2. Exhale and lift your legs, feet, head, and shoulders. Gaze across your legs to your toes. Lift through your chest and keep your back ribs on the floor. Either fold your arms and interlace your hands behind your head, or extend your arms toward your legs with your palms alongside your thighs. Breathe steadily.

3. Exhale to release from the pose. Bend your knees and lower your feet to the floor.

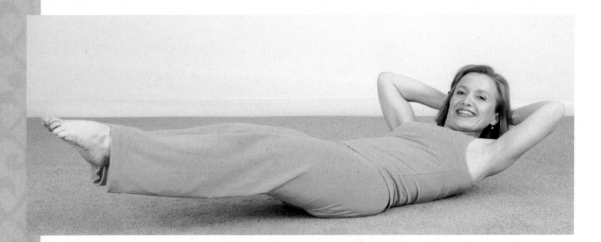

Gaze:	Center of the forehead
Warm-ups:	Warrior I (page 27), Sun Salutations (pages 76-79), Easy Sit-ups (page 21).
Counterposes:	Wind Reliever (page 48), Reclined Hip Rolls (page 54), Bridge Pose (page 64).
Easy variation:	Bend your knees; lean back on your elbows.
Benefits:	Tones the lower abdominal, leg, and back muscles.
Breathing:	Lie on your back on the floor. Inhale, lengthen and activate your body. Exhale, lift your upper body and legs. Exhale, lower your body to the floor.

FULL BOAT

1. Begin by sitting in Staff Pose (page 23) with both legs extended forward. Activate your legs. Place your feet together.

2. Lean back. Activate your abdominal muscles and move into a resting pose, with your legs lifted and bent and your calves parallel to the floor. Straighten your arms, bringing your palms alongside your thighs.

3. Exhale, straighten your legs, and lift your feet a little higher than your line of sight. Lift through your chest and straighten your back. Breathe steadily.

4. Exhale to release from the pose. Bend your knees and lower your feet to the floor.

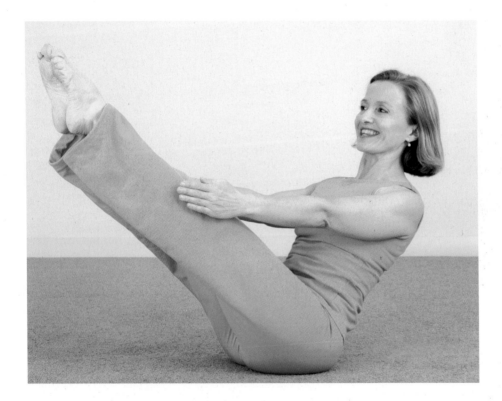

Gaze:	Center of the forehead.
Warm-ups:	Warrior I (page 27), Sun Salutations (pages 76-79), Easy Sit-ups (page 21).
Counterposes:	Wind Reliever (page 48), Reclined Hip Rolls (page 54), Bridge Pose (page 64).
Easy variation:	Bend your knees; lean back on your elbows.
Benefits:	Tones the upper abdominal, leg, and back muscles.
Breathing:	From Step 2: Inhale, lengthen your spine and activate your abdominal muscles. Exhale, extend your legs. Inhale, draw your knees back toward your shoulders. Exhale, lower your body into a sitting position.

HALF SPINAL TWIST

1. Begin by sitting with your legs crossed. Position your heel next to your right hip. Draw your right knee up in front of your chest and place your foot on the outside of your left knee. Position your right foot flat on the ground. Wrap your left arm around your right knee.

2. Inhale, lengthen your spine, and raise your right arm over your shoulder.

3. Exhale, twist to the right, and place your right hand behind your hip, keeping your fingertips out.

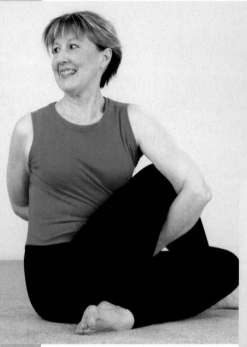

4. Inhale and release from the twist. Exhale and release your arms and legs. Repeat on the other side.

HALF SPINAL TWIST, LEG STRAIGHT

1. Practice the Half Spinal Twist (above) with the lower leg extended straight forward.

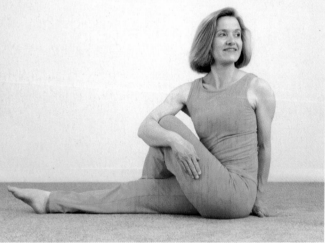

Gaze:	Over the shoulder.
Warm-ups:	Hip Spiral (page 53), Single Leg Forward Bend (page 43).
Counterposes:	Double Leg Forward Bend (page 42), Child's Pose (page 207), Shooting Star (page 200).
Easy variation:	Sit on a pillow; place one hand on the opposite knee to twist.
Benefits:	Excellent twist for the spine and massage for the internal organs; relieves stiffness in the lower back and hip joints.
Breathing:	Inhale, lengthen your spine. Exhale, twist. Inhale, release back to center. Exhale, release your arms and legs.

HIP SPIRAL

1. Begin by kneeling in the center of the yoga mat.
2. Exhale and shift your left hip to the floor. Stack your feet and ankles comfortably.
3. Inhale and lengthen your spine. Exhale and twist to the left, placing your right hand on your left thigh and your left hand behind your hip.
4. Inhale and release from the pose. Exhale and release your arms and legs. Repeat on the other side.

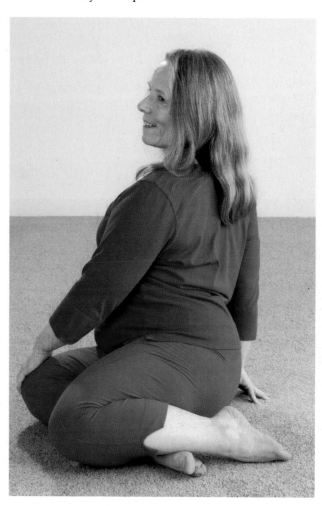

Gaze:	Over the shoulder.
Warm-ups:	Sitting Hip Rolls (page 199), Half Spinal Twist (page 52), Single Leg Forward Bend (page 43).
Counterposes:	Double Leg Forward Bend (page 42), Child's Pose (page 207), Shooting Star (page 200).
Easy variation:	Sit on a pillow.
Benefits:	Excellent twist for the spine and shoulders; relieves stiffness in the lower back.
Breathing:	Inhale, lengthen your spine. Exhale, twist. Inhale, release back to center. Exhale, release your arms and legs.

RECLINED HIP ROLLS

1. Begin by resting on the yoga mat with your knees bent. Position your arms on the floor in the T-position (page 23).

2. Inhale and raise your legs above your hips, keeping your knees bent.

3. Moving with your breath, exhale and roll your knees down to your left. Rotate your head to the right and gaze at your right hand.

4. Inhale and lift your knees back to center. Exhale and roll your knees to the other side.

5. Inhale and lift your knees back to center. Exhale and release your legs, stretching them out across the floor.

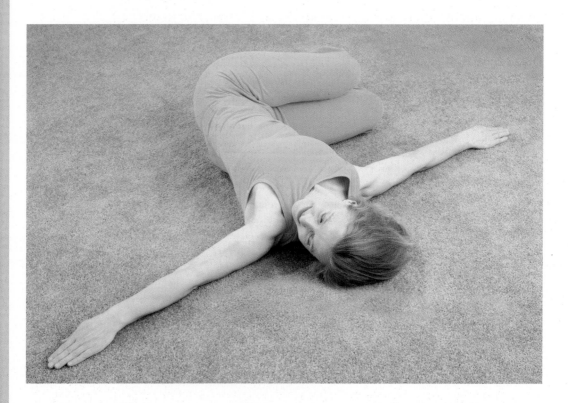

Gaze:	Hand opposite the legs in the twist.
Warm-ups:	Full Boat (page 51), Half Spinal Twist (page 52), Wind Reliever (page 48).
Counterposes:	Prop your legs against the wall; Double Leg Wind Reliever (page 48).
Easy variation:	Keep your toes on the floor.
Benefits:	Excellent twist for the spine and massage for the internal organs; relieves stiffness in the lower back and hip joints.
Breathing:	Inhale, lengthen your spine. Exhale, twist. Inhale, release back to center. Exhale, release your arms and legs.

HIP ROLLS WITH STRAIGHT LEGS

1. Begin by resting on the yoga mat with your legs straight. Position your arms on the floor in the T-position (page 23).

2. Inhale, activate your abdominal muscles, and raise your legs above your hips.

3. Moving with your breath, exhale, shift your hips to the right, and roll your legs down to the left. Rotate your head to the right and gaze at your right hand.

4. Inhale and lift your legs back to center. Repeat on the other side.

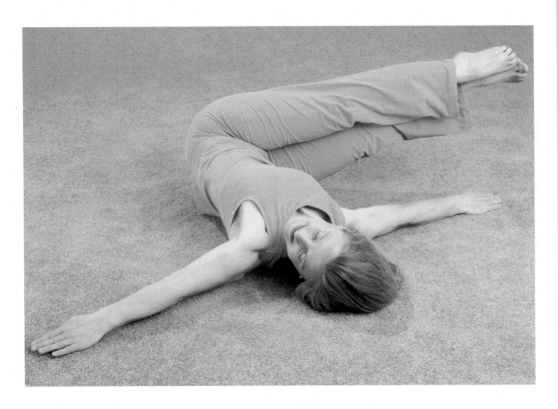

COBRA

1. Begin by lying on the yoga mat, face down. Activate your entire body and draw your heels in toward each other. Tighten your buttocks and slide your hands, palms down, underneath your shoulders. Spread your fingers out evenly and press down through your knuckles.

2. Inhale; keep your legs and buttocks tightened; and brush your forehead, nose, and chin across the floor and up. Lift your head and shoulders so that there is a gentle arch in your back. Keep your elbows in close to your sides and position your shoulders down and away from your ears.

3. Exhale, release from the pose, and stretch your arms down to your sides. Turn your head to one side.

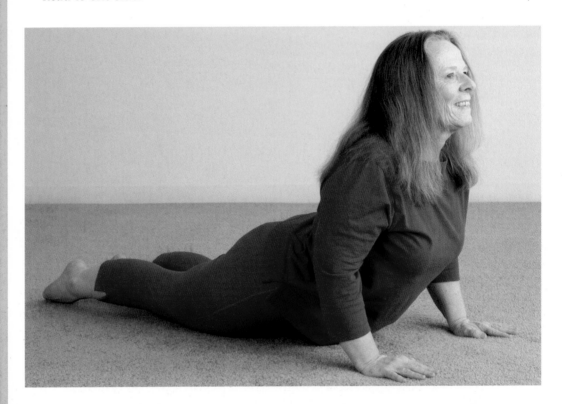

Gaze:	Center of the forehead.
Warm-ups:	Warrior I (page 27), Staff of Brahma (page 74), Sphinx (page 57).
Counterposes:	Devotional Pose (page 207), Downward Facing Dog (page 73).
Easy variation:	Sphinx (page 57).
Benefits:	Gentle massage for the spine; strengthens and tones the back muscles.
Breathing:	Inhale, lift your head and lengthen your spine. Exhale, release your upper body to the floor.

SPHINX

1. Begin by lying on the yoga mat, face down. Activate your entire body and draw your heels in toward each other. Tighten the buttocks and slide your forearms and elbows underneath your shoulders. Place your hands palms down and evenly spread your fingers.

2. Inhale; keep your legs and buttocks tightened; and brush your forehead, nose, and chin across the floor and up. Lift your head and shoulders so that there is a gentle arch in your back. Keep your elbows on the floor and in close to your sides. Position your shoulders down and away from your ears.

3. Exhale, release from the pose, and stretch your arms down to your sides. Turn your head to one side.

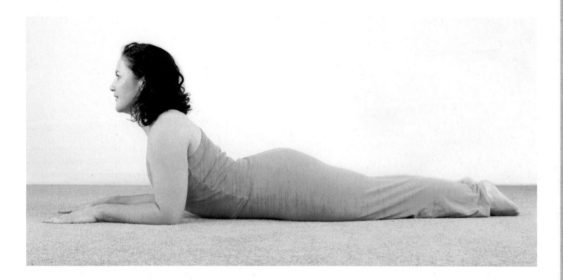

HALF LOCUST

1. Begin by lying on the yoga mat, face down. Activate your entire body and draw your heels in toward each other. Tighten your buttocks and slide your hands, palms down, underneath your hips. Position your elbows underneath your body and place your chin on the floor.

2. Inhale, keeping your legs and buttocks tightened, and lift your right leg as far as possible. Keep your right hip on the floor and your leg straight.

3. Exhale and release your leg. Repeat on the other side.

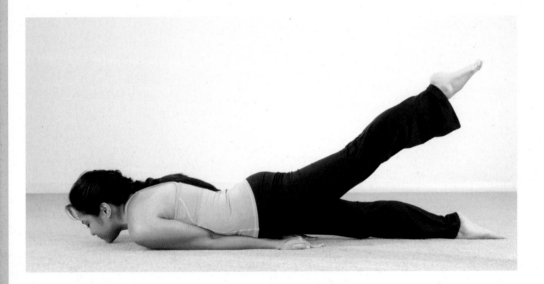

Gaze:	Center of the forehead.
Warm-ups:	Warrior III (page 34), Cobra (page 56).
Counterposes:	Devotional Pose (page 207), Downward Facing Dog (page 73).
Easy variation:	Stretch your arms forward and raise your right arm and left leg. Repeat on the other side.
Benefits:	Gentle massage for the spine; strengthens and tones the lower back muscles.
Breathing:	Inhale, lift your leg and lengthen your spine. Exhale, release your leg to the floor.

LOCUST

1. Begin by lying on the yoga mat, face down. Activate your entire body and draw your heels in toward each other. Tighten your buttocks. Roll your hands into fists and slide them, palms down, underneath your hips. Position your elbows underneath your body and place your chin on the floor.

2. Inhale, keeping your legs and buttocks tightened, and lift both legs as far as possible. Keep your hips on the floor and your legs straight.

3. Exhale and release your legs.

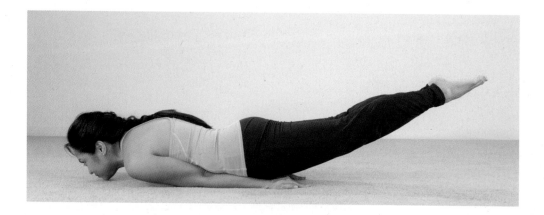

Gaze:	Center of the forehead.
Warm-ups:	Cobra (page 56), Half Bow (page 60).
Counterposes:	Devotional Pose (page 207), Downward Facing Dog (page 73.)
Easy variation:	Half Locust (page 58).
Benefits:	Gentle massage for the spine; strengthens and tones the lower back muscles.
Breathing:	Inhale, lift your legs and lengthen your spine. Exhale, release your legs to the floor.

HALF BOW

1. Begin by lying on your right side, stretched out in one plane on the yoga mat. Extend your lower arm straight forward, palm down and perpendicular to your body for balance. Bend your top leg and grasp the top side of your ankle with your left hand.

2. Inhale, arch, and raise your top leg and arm, with your foot being the highest point. Keep your hips squared but allow your top hip to drop forward enough so you can arch easily. Remain in the pose, breathing naturally.

3. Exhale and release from the pose. Lower your top arm and leg. Repeat on the other side.

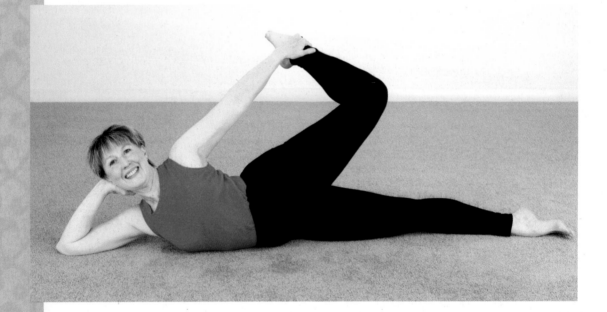

Gaze:	Center of the forehead.
Warm-ups:	Cobra (page 56), Locust (page 59).
Counterposes:	Devotional Pose (page 207), Wind Reliever (page 48).
Easy variation:	Rest your head on a pillow. Lift your top leg only a few inches.
Benefits:	Gentle massage for the spine; strengthens and tones the lower back and abdominal muscles.
Breathing:	Inhale, lift your top leg and lengthen your spine. Exhale, release your top leg to the floor.

BOW

1. Begin by lying face down on the yoga mat. Reach back to grasp both ankles. Keep your ankles and knees hip distance apart.

2. Inhale and pull against your ankles to lift easily into an arch. Lift your shoulders and chest and position your head with your chin parallel to the floor. Keep your legs hip distance apart. Breathe steadily.

3. Exhale and release from the pose. Relax in Devotional Pose (page 207).

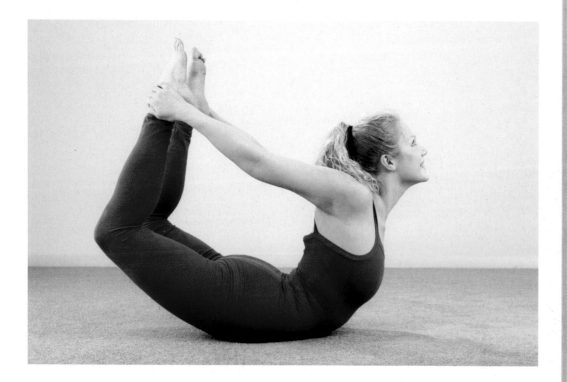

Gaze:	Center of the forehead.
Warm-ups:	Cobra (page 56), Half Bow (page 60).
Counterposes:	Devotional Pose (page 207), Double Leg Forward Bend (page 42), Shooting Star (page 200).
Easy variation:	Lying facedown, stretch one leg at a time by catching just one ankle and keeping the arch mild.
Benefits:	Strong massage for the spine; strengthens and tones the lower back and abdominal muscles.
Breathing:	Inhale, lift your legs and upper body. Exhale, release your legs and upper body to the floor.

CAMEL

1. Begin in an upright kneeling position. Place your knees and ankles hip distance apart. Tighten your buttocks.

2. Place your hands on your lower back. Inhale and lengthen your spine. Exhale and arch back, reaching your hands toward your heels. Position your hips over your knees. Relax your head back.

3. Keeping your hands on your lower back, inhale and lift your shoulders back up. Exhale and release into Devotional Pose (page 207).

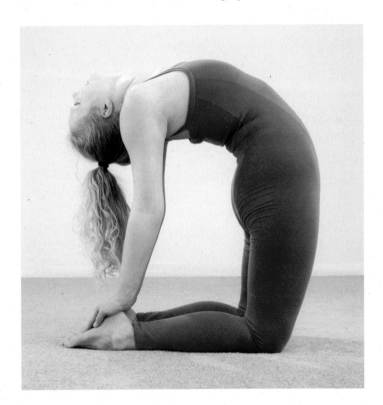

Gaze:	Center of the forehead.
Warm-ups:	Sun Salutations (pages 76-79), Crossbar (page 49), Cobra (page 56).
Counterposes:	Sitting Hip Rolls (page 199), Half Spinal Twist (page 52), Reverse Plank (page 165).
Easy variation:	Reach back for a chair; curl your toes under your heels.
Benefits:	Strong massage for the spine; strengthens and tones the lower back and abdominal and shoulder muscles.
Breathing:	Inhale, lengthen your spine. Exhale, arch in the pose while dropping your head back. Inhale, lift your head. Exhale, release into Devotional Pose (page 207).

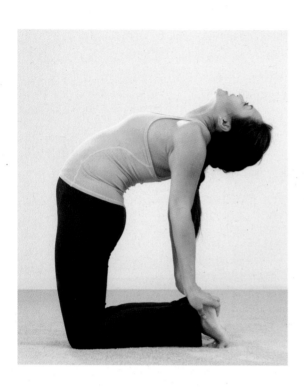

Camel with Toes Curled

1. Practice Camel (page 62) with your toes curled underneath your heels.

Camel with Chair

1. Practice Camel (page 62) reaching back for a chair seat.

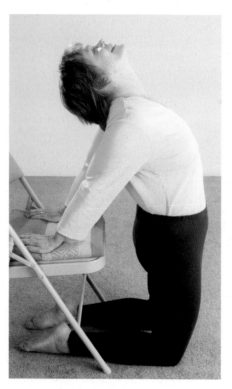

BRIDGE POSE

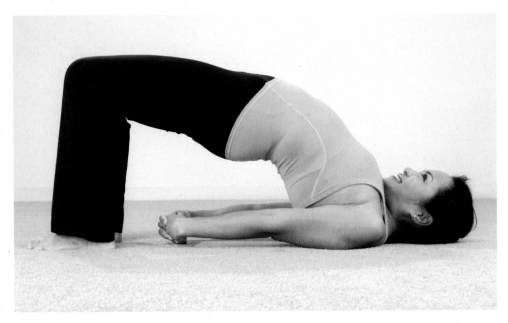

1. Begin by resting on the yoga mat face up. Activate your abdominal muscles. Bend both legs and place your feet parallel to each other underneath your knees.

2. Exhale and press your lower back to the floor. Tighten your buttocks, and inhale while lifting your hips. Draw your arms and shoulders underneath your body to support your hips. Place your hands under the boney crest of your hip. Extend fully in the pose, breathing steadily.

3. Exhale and release from the pose by gently placing each vertebra on the floor.

Gaze:	Center of the forehead.
Warm-ups:	Sun Salutations (pages 76-79), Warrior I (page 27), Half Spinal Twist (page 52).
Counterposes:	Hip Spiral (page 53), Wind Reliever (page 48).
Easy variation:	Place a pillow under your low back.
Benefits:	Strengthens and promotes flexibility for the spine.
Breathing:	Exhale, press your back to the floor. Inhale, lift your hips and spine. Exhale, release your hips and spine to the floor.

SIMPLE FISH

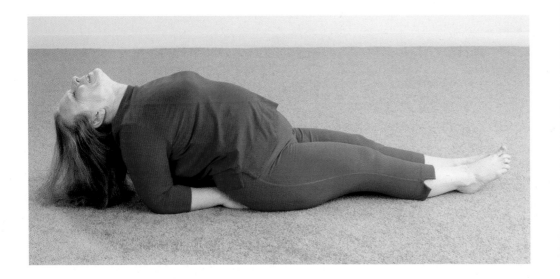

1. Begin by lying on your back on the yoga mat. Position your hands palms down, with your fingertips underneath your hips.

2. Inhale and lift up your head and torso to look at your toes.

3. Exhale and lean onto your elbows, dropping your head back. Position your elbows underneath your ribs. Draw your shoulder blades in toward your spine for support. Lift through your heart.

4. Inhale and lift your head to begin coming out of the pose. Exhale and lower your head and shoulders down to the floor. Release your hands to your sides.

Gaze:	Center of the forehead.
Warm-ups:	Bridge Pose (page 64), Reverse Plank (page 165), Half Bow (page 60).
Counterposes:	Wind Reliever (page 48), Supine Cross-Legged Twist (page 205).
Easy variation:	Lean your shoulders back over a cushion.
Benefits:	Strong massage for the neck and spine; strengthens and tones the lower back and abdominal muscles.
Breathing:	Inhale, lift your upper body up onto your elbows. Exhale, lower your head back. Inhale, lift your head up. Exhale, release your upper body to the floor.

65

HALF SUPINE HERO

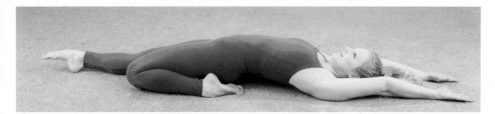

1. Begin by sitting in Staff Pose (page 23) with both legs stretched out and your feet together. Bring your lower left leg behind you, drawing your heel to your hip with your toes straight back. Activate your extended right leg and bring your knees in toward each other.

2. Exhale and lower your shoulders back toward the floor, keeping your knees on the floor. Rest on your elbows if your left knee begins to lift.

3. Inhale, lift your shoulders, and straighten your left leg. Sit in Staff Pose to switch sides. Repeat with your lower right leg in reverse.

SUPINE HERO WITH DOUBLE LEG

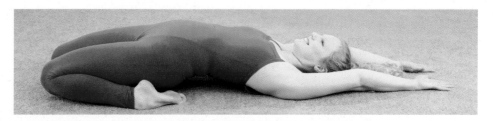

1. Begin kneeling with your hips on your heels. Then reposition your feet to the outsides of your legs with your heels to your hips and your toes straight back. Bring your knees in toward each other.

2. Exhale and lower your shoulders back, keeping your knees on the floor. Rest on your elbows if your knees begin to lift.

3. Inhale to come out of the pose, and lift your shoulders up using your arms for support. Exhale forward from the kneeling position into Devotional Pose (page 207).

Gaze:	Center of the forehead.
Warm-ups:	Quad Stretch at Wall (page 198), Single Leg Forward Bend (page 43), Bridge Pose (page 64).
Counterposes:	Devotional Pose (page 207), Double Leg Forward Bend (page 42).
Easy variation:	Lean back on cushions.
Benefits:	Strong massage for the spine and lower back; strengthens and tones the lower back, quadriceps, and abdominal muscles; increases circulation in the knee and ankle joints.
Breathing:	Inhale, lengthen your spine. Exhale, lower your back. Inhale, lift your upper body back. Exhale, stretch out your leg.

UPWARD FACING DOG

1. Begin in Devotional Pose (page 207).

2. Inhale and move forward and up, extending your back. Activate your entire body and draw your heels in toward each other. Tighten your buttocks and shift your hips forward toward the line of your wrists.

3. Position your hands, palms down, underneath your shoulders. Spread your fingers evenly and press down through your knuckles. Draw your shoulder blades down and back. Lift your head and chest, keeping your chin parallel to the floor.

4. Exhale, release your back, and relax in Devotional Pose (page 207).

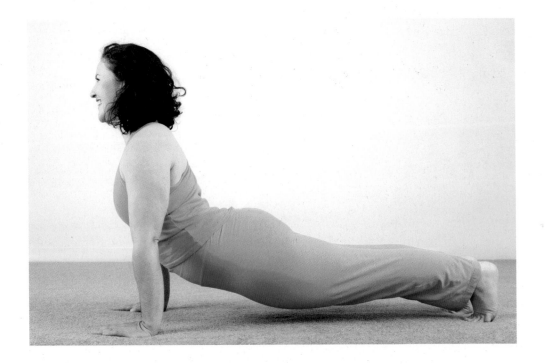

Gaze:	Center of the forehead.
Warm-ups:	Sun Salutations (pages 76-79), Cobra (page 56).
Counterposes:	Devotional Pose (page 207), Downward Facing Dog (page 73), Shooting Star (page 200).
Easy alternatives:	Cobra (page 56), Sphinx (page 57).
Easy variation:	Place a cushion underneath the hips.
Benefits:	Strong massage for the spine; strengthens and tones the upper body, lower back, and abdominal muscles.
Breathing:	Inhale, lift your upper body. Exhale, release back into Devotional Pose (page 207).

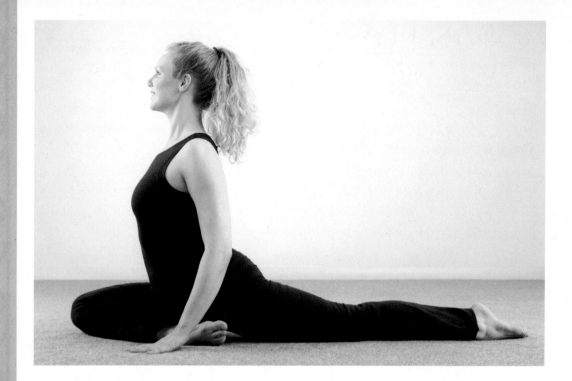

PIGEON POSE WITH ONE LEG EXTENDED

1. Begin by sitting with your legs crossed. With your hands on the yoga mat, shoulder distance apart, lean forward and place your right knee underneath your shoulders, with your right foot under your left hip. Stretch your left leg straight back, with your kneecap and top of your foot on the floor. Square your hips and tighten your left buttock.

2. Inhale, extend through the spine, and lift your chest and shoulders. Slide your hands to the sides of your hips for support. Activate your extended leg. Remain in the posture for four to six breaths, breathing fully and steadily.

3. Exhale to release from the back extension and rest in Devotional Pose (page 207). Repeat on the other side.

PIGEON POSE
WITH ONE LEG EXTENDED (RECLINED)

1. Come into Pigeon Pose with One Leg Extended (page 68) and exhale to relax forward. Lower your shoulders and stretch your arms forward, or cross your forearms underneath your head. Square your hips without leaning to one side for the best hip stretch.

2. Inhale and release from the pose. Lift your shoulders, using your arms for support. Exhale and rest in Devotional Pose (page 207). Repeat on the other side.

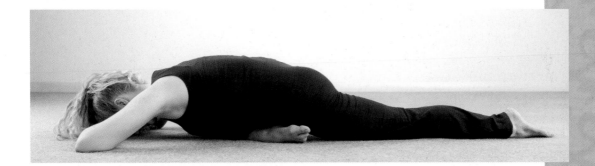

Gaze:	Center of the forehead.
Warm-ups:	Bridge Pose (page 64), Sitting Cradle Stretch (page 200), Half Lotus (page 89), Scissor Split (page 134), Upward Bow (page 128).
Counterposes:	Devotional Pose (page 207).
Easy variation:	Extend the back leg.
Benefits:	Tremendous opening for the shoulders, hips, and spine.
Breathing:	Inhale, extend your spine. Exhale, reach for your foot. Exhale, release from the pose.

SHOULDERSTAND

1. Begin by lying on the yoga mat face up. Prepare for the posture by resting your shoulders on a folded blanket. Exhale and roll your knees above your shoulders. Pause there to rotate your shoulders underneath your back. Interlace your fingers and bring your straight arms to the floor. Again, adjust your shoulders, rotating them in further.

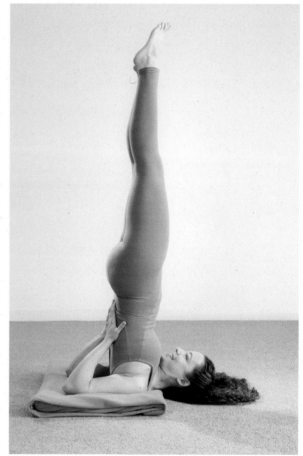

2. Release your hands and press them against your ribs to keep your torso vertical. Inhale and lift your legs into a vertical position over your shoulders. Pause here to adjust the pose. Press against your ribs to lift your torso straighter. Tuck in your pelvis. Activate your abdominal muscles and tighten your legs. Point your toes and bring your feet over your eyes.

3. Release from the pose by exhaling and lowering your legs. Release your hands to your sides. Inhale and roll out of the pose, returning to the floor.

Gaze:	Center of the forehead.
Warm-ups:	Bridge Pose (page 64), Simple Fish (page 65), Half Spinal Twist (page 52), Lunges (page 22), Scissor Split (page 134).
Counterposes:	Simple Fish (page 65), Wind Reliever (page 48), Supine Cross-Legged Twist (page 205).
Easy variation:	Walk your feet up the wall, and gently rotate to the left and to the right.
Benefits:	Massages the shoulders and stimulates the thyroid.
Breathing:	Exhale, roll your legs up above your shoulders. Inhale, lift your legs into a vertical position. Exhale, twist your legs and torso. Inhale, twist back to center. Exhale, roll out of the pose.

PLOW

1. Begin by lying on the yoga mat, face up. Rest your shoulders on a folded blanket. Exhale and roll your knees above your shoulders. Pause there to rotate your shoulders underneath your back.

2. Exhale and bring your toes all the way over your head to the floor.

3. Release from the pose by exhaling and lowering your legs to the yoga mat. Release your hands to your sides. Inhale and roll out of the pose, returning to the floor in Savasana (page 206).

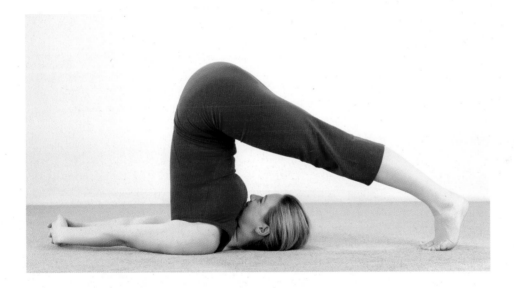

Gaze:	Center of the forehead.
Warm-ups:	Bridge Pose (page 64), Shoulderstand (page 70), Simple Fish (page 65), Half Spinal Twist (page 52), Lunges (page 22), Scissor Split (page 134).
Counterposes:	Simple Fish (page 65), Wind Reliever (page 48), Supine Cross-Legged Twist (page 205).
Easy variation:	Walk your feet up the wall, and gently rotate to the left and to the right.
Benefits:	Massages the shoulders, stimulates the thyroid, stretches the spine, and is a great warm up for Shoulderstand (page 70).
Breathing:	Exhale, roll your legs over your shoulders. On the next exhalation, begin rotating by walking your feet to one side. Inhale, rotate back to center. Exhale, roll your hips to the floor out of the pose. Inhale, lower your legs back to the mat in Savasana (page 206).

71

HEADSTAND

1. Begin in Devotional Pose (page 207). Position your elbows on the yoga mat a forearm's distance apart. Place your hands on the mat and interlace your fingers. Open the hands palms up and thumbs apart in order to rest the crown of your head in your hands. Your chin will be parallel to the mat in the pose.

2. Inhale and kick your legs straight up. This may be done with straight legs, either one leg raised at a time or with both legs raised together. Your legs may also be curled and slowly extended upward into the pose.

3. Activate your whole body. Lengthen up through your spine. Gently tuck your pelvis. Bring your ankles and heels together. Stretch up through the balls of your feet. Align your body vertically.

4. Exhale and release your legs down to come out of the pose. Remain in Devotional Pose (page 207) for four to six breaths in order to relax your breathing and heart rate.

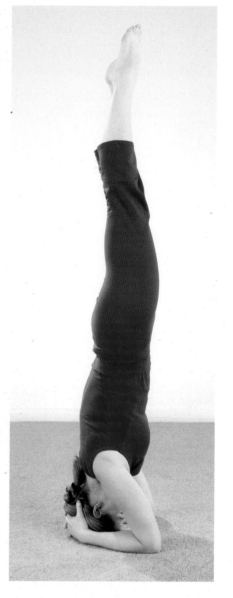

Gaze:	Center of the forehead.
Warm-ups:	Sun Salutations (pages 76-79).
Counterposes:	Devotional Pose (page 207), Shoulderstand (page 70), Simple Fish (page 65), Wind Reliever (page 48).
Easy variation:	Lift your hips only, without lifting your legs into the pose.
Benefits:	Strengthens and tones the whole body, and stimulates metabolism.
Breathing:	Exhale, lift your hips. Inhale, lift your legs. Exhale, release your legs to the floor.

DOWNWARD FACING DOG

1. Begin in Table Pose (page 23), with your toes curled under.
2. Exhale, lift your hips, and press down through your heels. Activate your thighs. Lift through your sit bones, and extend through your spine. Rotate your shoulder blades down and back toward your spine. Relax your head. Gaze at your knees.
3. Inhale and release into Table Pose (page 23). Exhale into Easy Sitting Pose (page 21).

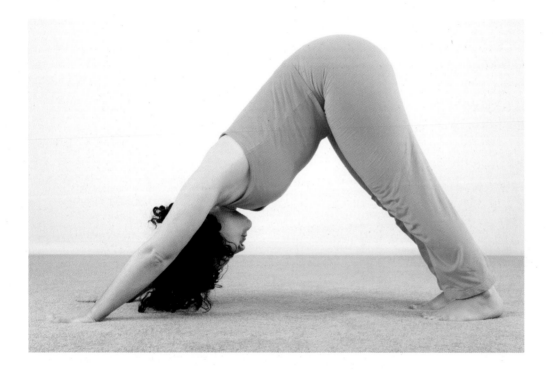

Gaze:	The knees or the center of the forehead.
Warm-ups:	Sun Salutations (page 76-79).
Counterposes:	Devotional Pose (page 207), Pigeon Pose with One Leg Extended (page 68).
Easy variation:	Bend your knees.
Benefits:	Builds upper body strength; hamstring stretch.
Breathing:	Exhale, press your hips up. Inhale, move back into Table Pose (page 23). Exhale, move into Easy Sitting Pose (page 21), with your legs crossed.

STAFF OF BRAHMA

1. Begin in Mountain (page 26) at the front end of the yoga mat. Bend your knees and keep your feet parallel, about three feet apart.

2. Inhale, with your palms together in front of your heart, straighten your legs, and reach up. Stretch your arms smoothly straight up and then out parallel to the floor, palms up.

3. Exhale and bend forward until your back and arms are parallel to the floor.

4. Inhale and stretch your arms over your shoulders, bringing your arms next to your ears. Rotate your palms toward each other.

5. Exhale, bend your knees, and round your back forward, placing your palms on the floor.

6. Inhale and roll up to a standing position, stretching your arms overhead.

7. Exhale, bend your knees, and bring your hands together in front of your heart.

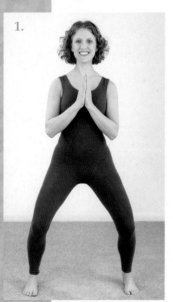

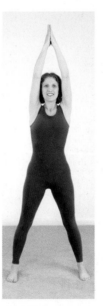

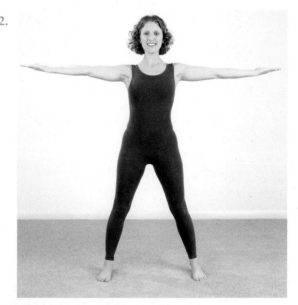

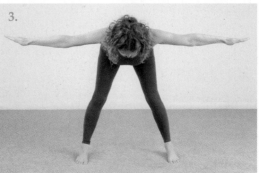

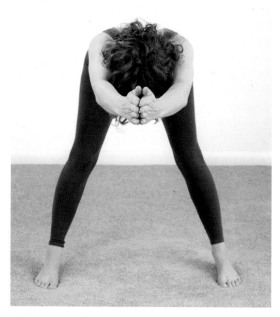

4.

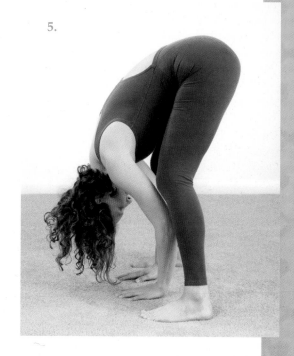

5.

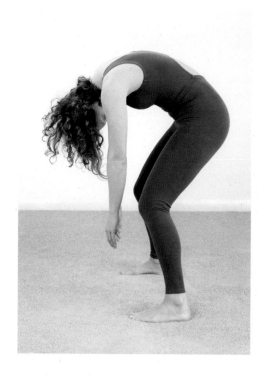

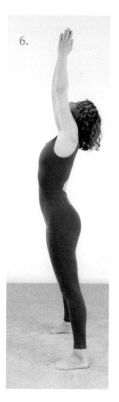

6.

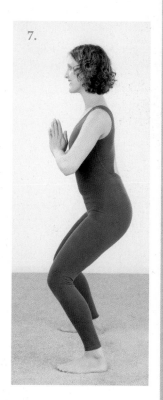

7.

SUN SALUTATION (EASY)

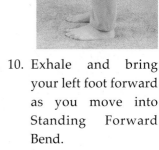

1.

1. Begin in Mountain (page 26) at the front end of the yoga mat.
2. Inhale, extend up, and arch into Crescent Stretch.
3. Exhale and bend forward, with your hips over your heels.
4. Inhale and step your right foot back into Lunge.
5. Retain your breath as you move into Plank.
6. Exhale and lower into Devotional Pose.
7. Inhale and extend forward into Cobra Pose, with your hands underneath your shoulders.
8. Exhale and lift your hips into Downward Facing Dog.
9. Inhale and bring your right foot forward, placing it between both hands.

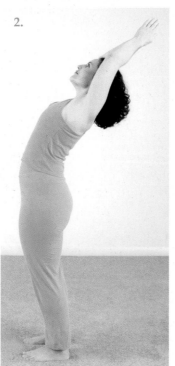

2.

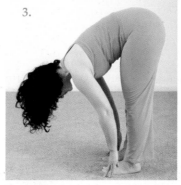

3.

4.

10. Exhale and bring your left foot forward as you move into Standing Forward Bend.

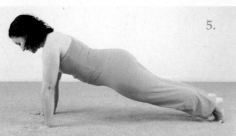

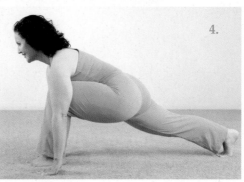

5.

11. Inhale, lift your shoulders, move into a standing position, and arch into Crescent Stretch.
12. Exhale and stand in Mountain (page 26).

6.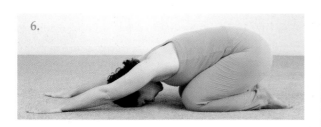

7.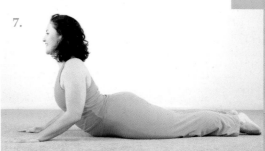

8.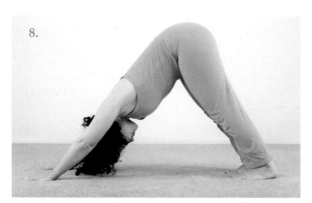

9.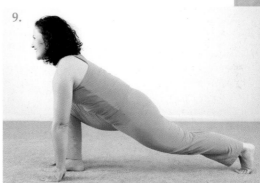

10.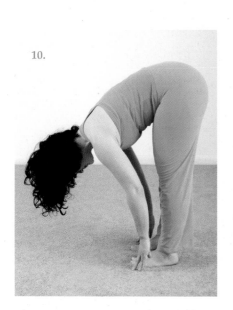

11.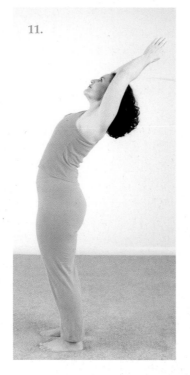

12.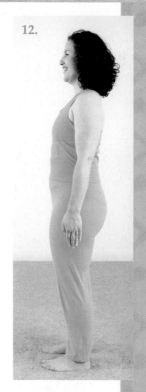

SUN SALUTATION (AEROBIC)

1. Begin in Mountain (page 26) at the front end of the yoga mat.
2. Inhale, extend up, and arch into Crescent Stretch.
3. Exhale and bend forward, with your hips over your heels.
4. Inhale and jump back into Plank.
5. Exhale and lower into Devotional Pose.
6. Inhale and extend forward into Upward Facing Dog.
7. Exhale and lift your hips into Downward Facing Dog.
8. Inhale and jump forward, placing both feet between both hands.
9. Exhale and lift your hips into Standing Forward Bend.
10. Inhale, lift your shoulders back until you are standing, and arch into Crescent Stretch.
11. Exhale and stand in Mountain (page 26).

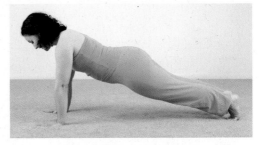

1.

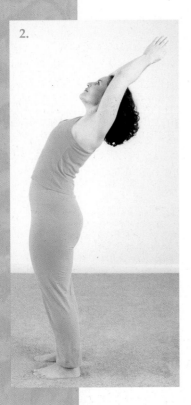

2.

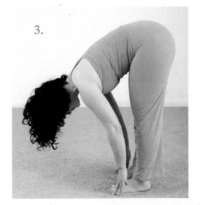

3.

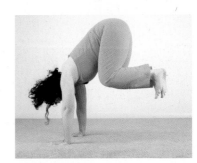

4.

78

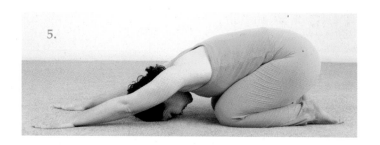

5.

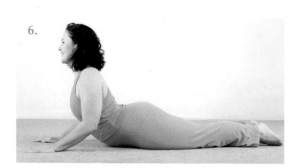

6.

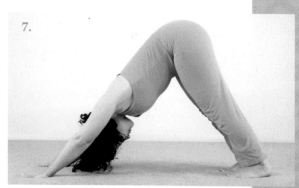

7.

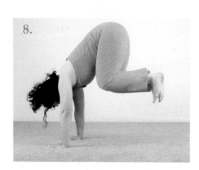

8.

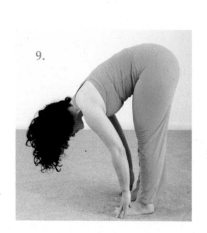

9.

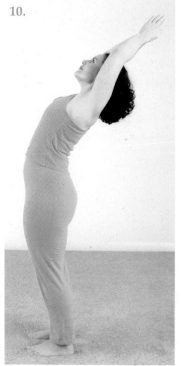

10.

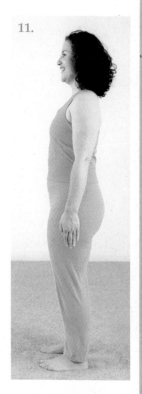

11.

MOON SALUTATION

1. Begin in Mountain (page 26) in the center of the yoga mat and take a step to each side so your feet are a leg's distance apart.

2. Inhale and raise your arms so they are parallel to the floor. Rotate your right foot out ninety degrees and your left foot in thirty degrees.

3. Exhale and bend right into Triangle.

4. Inhale and lunge by bending your right leg. Place your right hand on the floor inside of your foot. Raise your left arm straight up.

5. On the next inhalation, raise your left leg for Half Moon. Press up through your left ankle bone. Straighten your right leg, which is supporting you. Reach straight up with your left arm.

6. Exhale and roll into Lunge, lowering your left foot to the floor. Place your hands on either side of your right foot.

7. Inhale, lower your left knee to the floor, and raise your arms above your shoulders, aligning them with your ears.

8. Exhale and lower your hands to your heart.

9. Inhale and extend your arms parallel to the floor. Exhale and twist to the left.

10. Inhale, release back to center, and place your hands on either side of your right foot.

11. Exhale and lower yourself into this variation of Single Leg Forward Bend. Fold your left leg. Bring your tailbone to your left heel. Bend forward over your extended right leg, keeping your head, neck, and spine aligned.

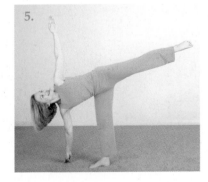

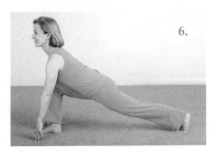

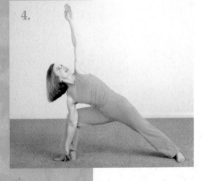

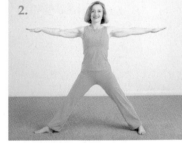

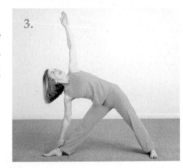

12. Inhale, place your hands on each side of your right leg, and lift into Lunge.

13. Exhale, rotate your hips and shoulders to the side, and place your left foot on the floor.

14. Inhale and lift into modified Lateral Angle.

15. On the next inhalation, lift into Warrior II.

16. On the next inhalation, lift into Standing Straddle.

17. Exhale into Mountain (page 26).

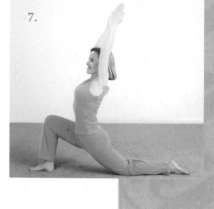

7.

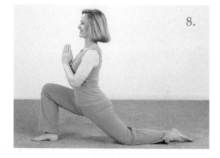

8.

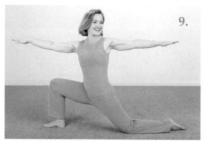

9.

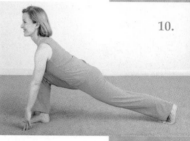

10.

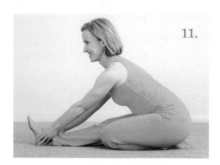

11.

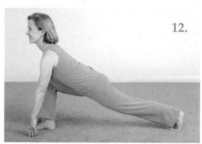

12.

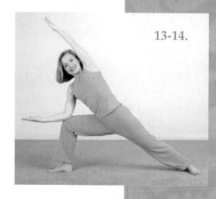

13-14.

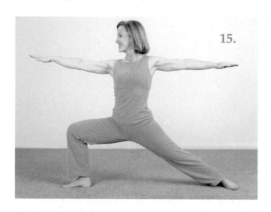

15.

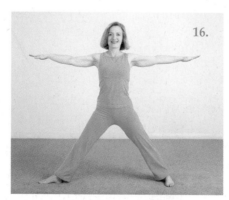

16.

Home Practice Sequences

Abdominal Breathing

This breathing style helps to ground you and may be combined with your yoga postures. Sit comfortably and rest your hands, palms down, on the knees. Breathe deeply so that your abdomen and torso expand with the inhalation and contract with the exhalation. Feel as though your abdominal muscles are the bellows for your breath. Inwardly, focus on the energy center just below your navel. Practicing abdominal-style breathing promotes feelings of confidence and well-being. It can help stabilize those who struggle with anxiety.

Ujjayi Breath

"Ujjayi" literally means victorious and refers to the upward movement of prana through the sushumna, or central channel. Ujjayi breathing is characterized by a steady and even flow. Normally the breath is slightly erratic; the inhalation or exhalation often begins quickly and ends slowly with less force. Ujjayi breathing provides a continuous flow without fluctuations. Slowly and continuously inhale with the same gentle constriction at the throat. Exhale in the same manner for an equal length of time. Do not create tension or harshness in the throat area. The breath sound should be soft and pleasing, never grating or strained.

Breath Awareness Meditation

How you approach meditation is very important. The more reverence you bring and the more sacred you make your time and space, the more sacredness you'll experience. Sit comfortably with your back straight, shoulders above your hips, and your hands resting on your thighs. Close your eyes and turn your attention inward. Notice your breathing. Where does it start? Where does it go inside? How does it feel? Is it fast or slow? What happens to your body when you breathe out? Where does your breath go? Continue to notice the qualities of your breath. You don't have to do anything to change it; just notice it. Get in touch with the flow of your breath; follow it as it moves in and out. There's no right way to feel, and there's nothing you have to do at this moment except watch the flow of your breath. Watch and feel the breath as it comes into your nose, through your throat, and into your chest. You may feel your diaphragm fill with air and your belly expanding with the breath. Watch and feel your breath as it flows out again from your lungs, through your throat, and out from your nose. Notice that as you begin to relax, your whole body just releases toward the floor. Let yourself soften from the inside out, but keep your back straight. As you relax, you may notice that your breath naturally becomes more relaxed and full. Even though you feel relaxed, keep your mind alert. By watching your breath, you can become even more relaxed than if you were asleep. It's okay if your attention should wander. Just bring your focus back to your breath. It really doesn't matter how many times your mind drifts away from the breath; what's important is that you keep bringing your mind back to your breathing.

Hatha Yoga Practice Sequences

Practice Sequence One

Mountain (Tadasana), page 26

Warrior I (Virabhadrasana I), page 27

Warrior II (Virabhadrasana II), page 28

Triangle (Trikonasana), page 30

Tree (Vrksasana), pages 32-33

Crescent Stretch, page 21

Standing Forward Bend (Uttanasana), page 37

Table Pose, page 23

Cat-Cow, page 198

Single Leg Forward Bend (Janu Sirsasana), page 43

Double Leg Forward Bend (Pascimottanasana), page 42

Bridge Pose (Setu Bandha Sarvangasana), page 64

Wind Reliever (Pavanamuktasana), page 48

Reclined Hip Rolls (Jathara Parivartanasana), pages 54-55

Savasana, page 206

Practice Sequence Two

Mountain (Tadasana), page 26

Easy Sun Salutation (Surya Namaskar), pages 76-77

Warrior I (Virabhadrasana I), page 27

Standing Head to Knee (Parsvottanasana), pages 39-41

Warrior II (Virabhadrasana II), page 28

Warrior III (Virabhadrasana III), page 34

Standing Forward Bend (Uttanasana), page 37

Practice Sequence Three

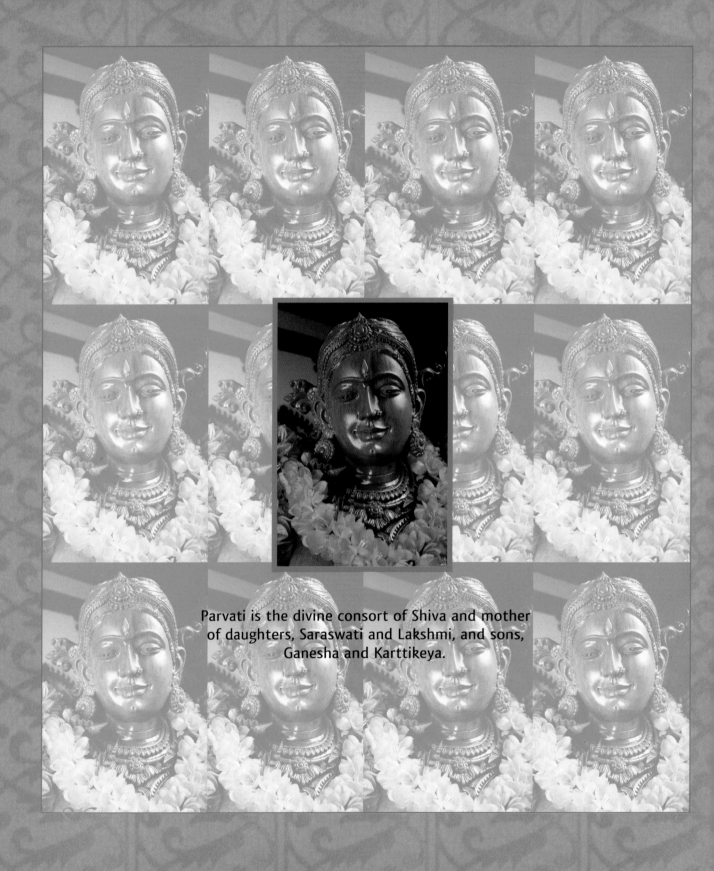

Parvati is the divine consort of Shiva and mother of daughters, Saraswati and Lakshmi, and sons, Ganesha and Karttikeya.

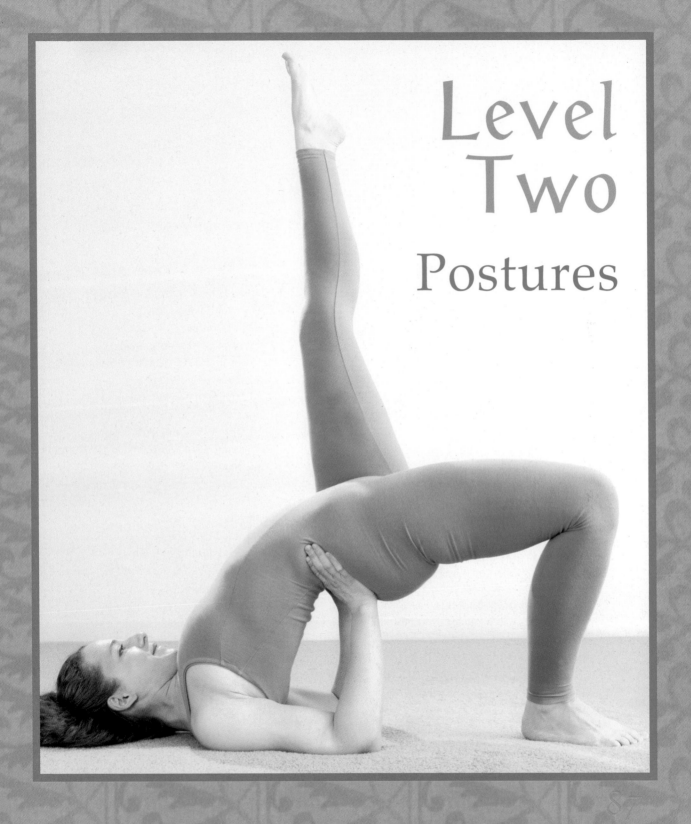

Level Two

Postures

Chapter Two

Level Two Postures

*"Enjoy the world, have your heaven even here on earth
while you are alive." – Faith Stone*

HALF LOTUS

1. Begin by sitting with your legs crossed. Draw your right foot up, with the heel toward your abdomen, and rest it on your left thigh. Position your foot close to your hip joint. The top arch of your foot or the ankle can rest on your left thigh.

2. Draw your sit bones back and slightly to the sides, allowing your right knee to relax to the floor. Gently rotate your skin and muscle on your right thigh and calf in order for your leg to settle into the posture.

3. To release, grasp your right ankle and lift your foot from your left thigh back to the floor. Repeat on your left side.

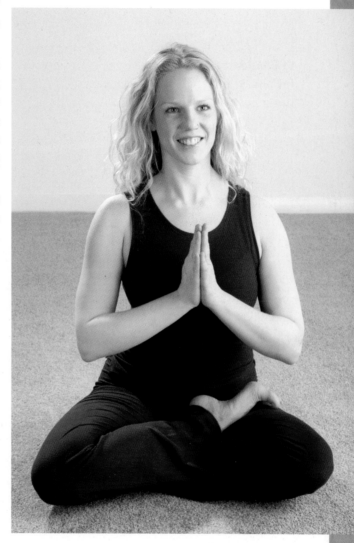

Gaze: Center of the forehead.
Warm-ups: Sitting Cradle Stretch (page 200), Single Leg Forward Bend (page 43).
Counterposes: Supine Crossed-Legged Twist (page 205), Wind Reliever (page 48).
Easy variation: Place a pillow under the elevated knee, sit on a cushion.
Benefits: Increases hip flexibility, keeps spine strong.
Breathing: Steady, even, full.

FULL LOTUS

1. Begin in the Easy Sitting Pose (page 21). Draw your right foot up, with the heel toward your abdomen, and rest it on your left thigh. Keep the foot snug against your hip joint. The top arch of your foot can rest on your left thigh or, if it's more comfortable, the ankle can rest on your thigh.

2. Draw your sit bones back and slightly to your sides, allowing your right knee to relax to the floor. Gently rotate the skin and muscle on your right thigh and calf in order for your leg to settle into the posture.

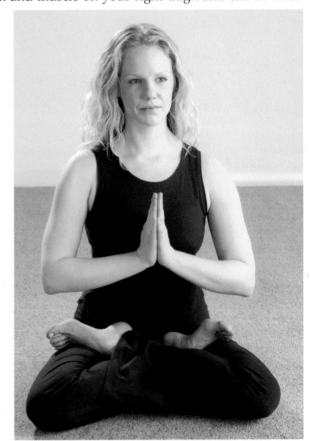

3. Draw your left foot up to rest on your right thigh, keeping it snug against your hip. Adjust your sit bones again for comfort.

4. Lift your shoulders, upper chest, and back ribs, creating a balanced sitting posture with the feeling of expansion going up your spine, through your heart, and up your back ribs. Your breath should remain full and steady. Keep your chin parallel to the floor and your ears over your shoulders. Smile gently to relax your face, neck, and collarbone area.

5. To release, grasp your right ankle and lift your foot from your left thigh back to the floor. Repeat on your left side.

Gaze:	Center of the forehead.
Warm-ups:	Sitting Cradle Stretch (page 200), Cat-Cow (page 198), Cow Face Pose (page 101).
Counterposes:	Single Leg Forward Bend (page 43), Sitting Hip Rolls (page 199).
Easy variation:	Use a pillow under the elevated knee; sit on a pillow.
Benefits:	Increases hip flexibility and circulation.
Breathing:	Steady, even, full.

STANDING LEG EXTENSION

1. Begin in Mountain (page 26) at the front end of the yoga mat. Draw your right knee up and grasp your big toe with the first two fingers of your right hand. Exhale and extend your right leg forward and up. Alternatively, interlace both hands around your heel. With your leg extended, draw it closer by bending your elbows.

2. To release from the pose, inhale and draw your knee to your chest. Exhale to return your right foot to the floor.

3. Repeat on your left side.

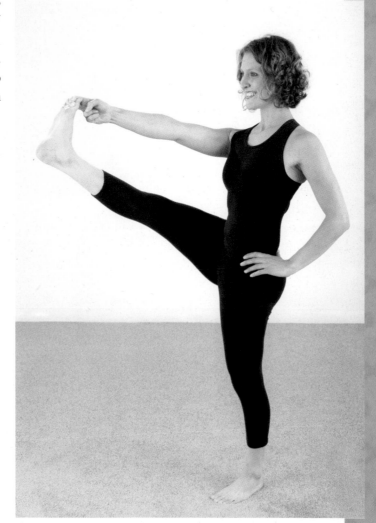

Gaze:	Big toe of the extended leg or the center of the forehead.
Warm-ups:	Standing Hip Stretches (page 23), Standing Forward Bend (page 37).
Counterposes:	Twisting Bear (page 197), Standing Forward Bend (page 37).
Easy variation:	Use a belt to assist the leg extension.
Benefits:	Greatly stretches the hips and hamstrings.
Breathing:	Exhale, extend your leg. Inhale, bring your knee back to your chest. Exhale, release your foot back to the floor.

STANDING CRADLE

1. Begin in Mountain (page 26) at the front end of the yoga mat. Draw your right knee up and cradle the lower right leg between both elbows. Straighten your spine, hugging the lower right leg toward your chest.

2. To release, exhale and return your right foot to the floor.

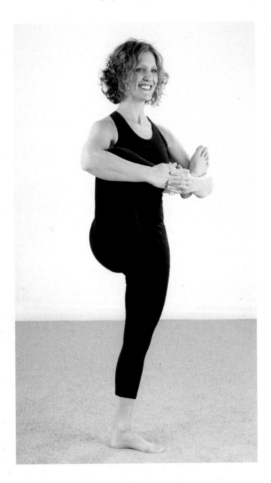

Gaze:	Center of the forehead.
Warm-ups:	Standing Hip Stretches (page 23), Standing Forward Bend (page 37).
Counterposes:	Twisting Bear (page 197), Standing Straddle Forward Bend (page 38).
Easy variation:	Begin with the Sitting Cradle Stretch (page 200).
Benefits:	Greatly stretches the hips and hamstrings.
Breathing:	Exhale, extend your leg. Inhale, bring knee to your chest. Exhale, release your foot back to the floor.

STANDING BOUND HALF LOTUS FORWARD BEND

1. Begin in Mountain (page 26) at the front end of the yoga mat. Shift your weight onto your right leg. Tuck in your pelvis. Lift your left leg into Half Lotus (page 89). Reach your left arm behind your hip to grasp your left foot.

2. Inhale and extend through your spine. Exhale into a forward bend, lifting your sit bones and keeping the supporting leg straight. Tighten your abdominal muscles. Reach your right hand toward the floor beside your right foot.

3. Breathe steadily in the pose.

4. To release from the pose, inhale and lift your torso and shoulders back to standing. Exhale and release your left foot to the floor.

5. Repeat on the other side.

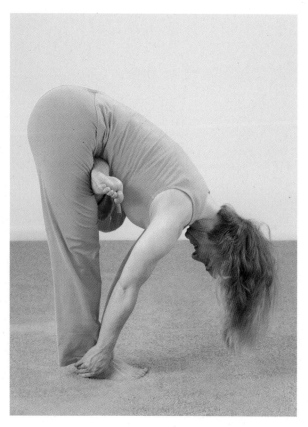

Gaze:	Center of the forehead or support foot.
Warm-ups:	Sitting Cradle Stretch (page 200), Standing Forward Bend (page 37), Half Spinal Twist (page 52).
Counterposes:	Standing Forward Bend (page 37), Chair (page 123).
Easy variation:	Single Leg Forward Bend (page 43).
Benefits:	Deep hip stretch and hamstring stretch; brings clear inner focus.
Breathing:	Inhale, extend your spine while standing. Exhale into a forward bend. Inhale, lift up. Exhale, release from the pose, foot to the floor.

LOTUS HAND BALANCE

1. Begin in Full Lotus (page 90). Place your hands palms down beside your hips. Inhale and lift your knees to activate your abdominal muscles. Exhale, keep the abdominal muscles tightened, and lift up. Keep your chest and head open and lifted.

2. Stay in the pose, breathing steadily, for four to six breaths.

3. To release from the pose, exhale and lower yourself back to the mat.

4. Reverse the cross on your legs and repeat.

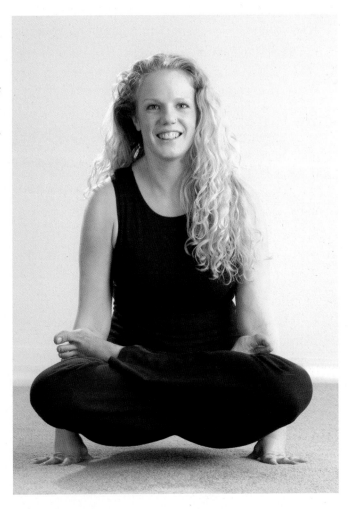

Gaze:	Center of the forehead.
Warm-ups:	Sitting Cradle Stretch (page 200), Half Lotus (page 89).
Counterposes:	Half Spinal Twist (page 52), Single Leg Forward Bend (page 43), Supine Cross-Legged Twist (page 205).
Easy variation:	Place yours fists or fingertips on the mat; try starting in Half Lotus (page 89) or sitting with your legs crossed.
Benefits:	Tones the abdominal muscles, improves digestion, builds upper body strength; strong hip stretch.
Breathing:	Steady and even.

LION POSE

1. Begin in Full Lotus (page 90). Inhale, lengthen your spine, and reach forward into a modified Table Pose (page 23). Exhale and lower your hips into an Upward Facing Dog (page 67) extension. Lift in your shoulders and heart.

2. Exhale, extend your tongue down to your chin, and roll your eyes, slightly crossing them and looking up. Stay in this extension for one more breath. Then exhale and release back to Full Lotus (page 90).

3. Recross your legs to switch sides in Full Lotus (page 90), and repeat.

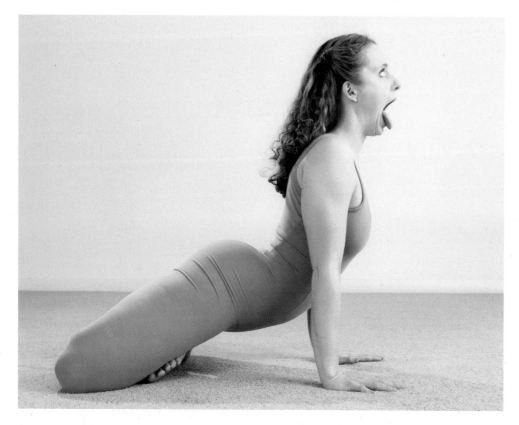

Gaze:	Center of the forehead.
Warm-ups:	Sitting Cradle Stretch (page 200), Half Lotus (page 89), Cat-Cow (page 198), Upward Facing Dog (page 67).
Counterposes:	Sitting Hip Roll (page 199), Downward Facing Dog (page 73).
Easy variation:	Do this posture either kneeling, sitting with your legs crossed, or in Half Lotus (page 89).
Benefits:	Tones the back and shoulders, promotes hip flexibility, releases toxins; good for the liver and kidneys.
Breathing:	From Full Lotus, inhale into Table. Exhale into an Upward Facing Dog extension. Inhale back into Table. Exhale into Full Lotus.

HIDDEN LOTUS

1. Begin in Full Lotus (page 90), with your left leg crossed over your right leg.

2. Breathe deeply and roll forward into a modified Table Pose (page 23).

3. Exhale and slowly lower yourself forward and down to the floor. Place your abdomen on the floor, with your hands out to your sides. Make sure that your feet are tucked comfortably underneath your body. Reach your right hand behind your back to catch your left wrist. Breathe deeply, with your chin resting on the floor.

4. Inhale, release your hands, and push up to a sitting position. Exhale and unfold your legs. Repeat on the other side.

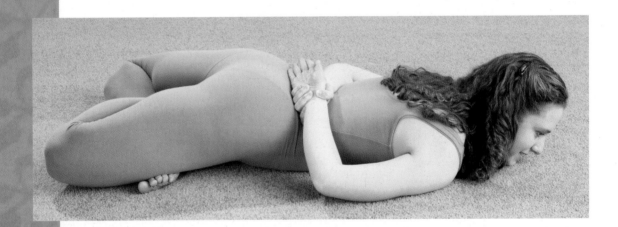

Gaze:	Center of the forehead.
Warm-ups:	Sitting Cradle Stretch (page 200), Half Lotus (page 89), Pigeon Pose with One Leg Extended (page 68).
Counterposes:	Half Spinal Twist (page 52), Wind Reliever (page 48).
Easy variation:	Use the Half Lotus (page 89) pose instead of the Full Lotus pose.
Benefits:	Calms the nerves and soothes emotions; strong hip stretch promotes back flexibility.
Breathing:	Inhale into modified Table Pose (page 23), Exhale, lower onto the mat. Remain in the pose four to six breaths. Inhale back into a sitting pose.

REVOLVED HALF MOON

1. Begin in Mountain (page 26) at the front end of the yoga mat. Exhale into Standing Forward Bend (page 37). Place both hands on the floor. Inhale, extend your right leg up and parallel to the floor, keeping your hips square to the floor.

2. Exhale and rotate your torso evenly to the left. Extend your left arm up above your shoulder, keeping your right leg parallel to the floor. Your right hip will rotate toward the floor as your entire spine twists. Rotate your head to look up at your left hand.

3. Release with an exhalation, lowering your left arm and right leg into a Standing Forward Bend. Inhale, lift your shoulders into Mountain (page 26). Repeat on the other side.

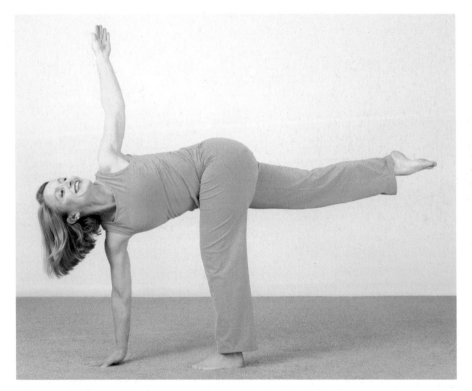

Gaze:	Top hand.
Warm-ups:	Triangle (page 30), Revolved Triangle (page 31), Lateral Angle (page 29), Revolved Lateral Angle (page 98).
Counterposes:	Standing Forward Bend (page 37), Standing Straddle Forward Bend (page 38), Twisting Bear (page 197).
Easy variation:	Drop your back knee to the floor in the revolved lateral angle.
Benefits:	Invigorating.
Breathing:	Exhale into Warrior II (page 28). Inhale, extend leg. Exhale into twist. Inhale, raise top arm and look up. Exhale down into a forward bend. Inhale into Mountain (page 26).

REVOLVED LATERAL ANGLE

1. Begin in a lunge with your right leg extended back. Drop your right heel to the mat. Bring your palms together in front of your heart and exhale while rotating to the left. Drop your right elbow to the outside of your left knee.

2. Extend your left arm and hand over your head, making a lateral extension from your left heel, hip, and shoulder to your left hand. Rotate your head to look up.

3. Exhale to release from the pose.

4. Repeat on the other side.

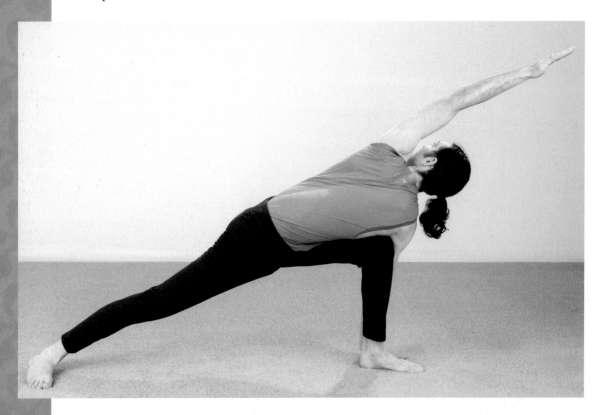

Gaze:	Look up.
Warm-ups:	Triangle (page 30), Revolved Triangle (page 31), Half Moon (page 36), Revolved Half Moon (page 97), Pigeon Pose with One Leg Extended (page 68).
Counterposes:	Standing Forward Bend (page 37), Standing Straddle Forward Bend (page 38), Sun Salutations (pages 76-79).
Easy variation:	In a lunge, just twist and rest your lower arm on your front thigh.
Benefits:	Good for digestion; strengthens and increases flexibility in legs, hips, back, and shoulders.
Breathing:	Exhale into twist. Inhale, extend arm overhead. Exhale, release from pose.

SINGLE LEG FORWARD BEND WITH HALF LOTUS

1. Begin in Easy Sitting Pose (page 21) and extend your left leg out straight. Make it strong and active. Push through the ball of your left foot.

2. Draw your right foot up, heel to abdomen, and rest it on your left thigh, drawing it up to your hip joint. The top arch of your foot can rest on your left thigh or, if it is more comfortable, your ankle can rest on your thigh.

3. Draw your sit bones back and slightly to the sides, allowing your right knee to relax to the floor. Gently rotate the skin and muscle on your right thigh and calf in order for your leg to settle into the posture.

4. Reach your right hand behind your back to catch your right foot. Inhale and lengthen your spine, extending the left arm overhead. Exhale into a forward bend, keeping your spine and shoulders aligned.

5. Inhale to come out of the pose, lifting your left arm over your shoulder. Exhale and release both arms and legs back into Staff Pose.

6. Repeat on the other side.

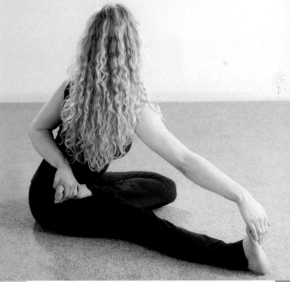

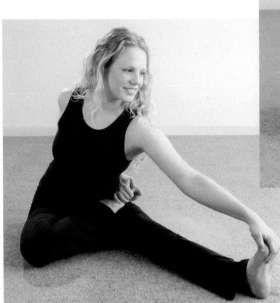

HIP SPIRAL WITH HALF LOTUS

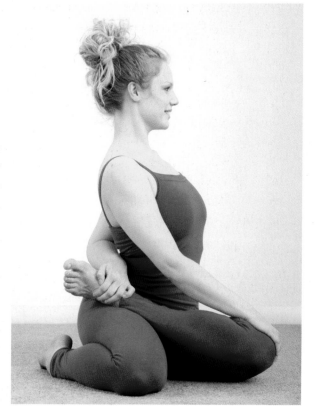

1. Begin kneeling. Exhale and drop your hips to the left. Draw your left foot up in the half lotus position. Reach your left hand behind your back to grasp your left foot. Exhale, twist your torso to the left. Inhale, lengthen your spine. Exhale, in the twist turn your head to look right.

2. Release from the pose. Inhale and relax back to center. Lower your left leg to the floor. Switch sides.

Gaze:	Gaze over your shoulder.
Warm-ups:	Sitting Cradle Stretch (page 200), Half Lotus (page 89), Half Spinal Twist (page 52).
Counterposes:	Shooting Star (page 200), Standing Forward Bend (page 37).
Benefits:	Excellent twist for the spine and massage for the internal organs; relieves stiffness in lower back and hip joints.
Breathing:	Inhale, lengthen your spine. Exhale, rotate and reach forward. Inhale to release. Exhale and relax.

COW FACE POSE

1. Begin sitting with your legs crossed. Cross your right leg over your left, aligning your knees. Adjust your legs so your heels are equal distance from your hips on both sides.

2. Inhale and stretch your right arm over your shoulder. Exhale and drop your right hand behind your back. Position your left arm behind your lower back, and catch your hands behind your back between your shoulder blades. If you prefer, hold a strap with your right hand while your left hand grasps the strap below.

Gaze:	Center of the forehead.
Warm-ups:	Sitting Cradle Stretch (page 200), Supine Hero (page 66).
Counterposes:	Forward Bends (see index), Shooting Star (page 200), and simple twists.
Easy variation:	Sit on a cushion. Try twisting in the pose.
Benefits:	Greatly stretches hips; increases circulation in ankles and knees and hips.
Breathing:	Steady, full, and even.

BRIDGE WITH HALF LOTUS

1. Begin resting on the mat face up. Activate your abdominal muscles and draw your right foot up. Place it in Half Lotus (page 89), resting it at the top of your left thigh. Bend your left leg to place your left foot on the mat. Move it a few inches toward the centerline of your body so it will be easier to balance.

2. Exhale, press your lower back to the mat. Tone your buttocks and inhale, lifting your hips. Draw your arms and shoulders underneath your body to support your hips, and place your hands under the boney crest of your hip. Extend fully in the pose, breathing steadily. This is a nice stretch for your hip.

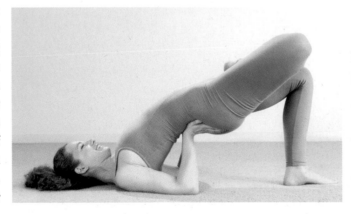

3. Exhale, release from the pose by gently releasing your vertebrae to the mat. Switch half lotus legs and repeat the pose on the other side. An alternative is to extend the half lotus leg straight up before releasing from the pose.

BRIDGE WITH LEG EXTENSION

1. Begin on the mat, face up. Activate your abdominal muscles. Place both feet on the mat as close to your hips as possible.

2. Exhale, press your low back to the mat. Tone your buttocks and inhale, lifting your hips. Draw your arms and shoulders underneath your body. To support your hips, place your hands under the boney crest of your hip, palms up.

3. Inhale, bend your right knee and draw it up above your hip, then straighten your leg and point your toes. The extended leg will be perpendicular to the mat. Breathing steadily, extend fully through your spine.

4. Exhale, release your extended leg so that your foot returns to the mat. Release your spine. Switch sides and repeat.

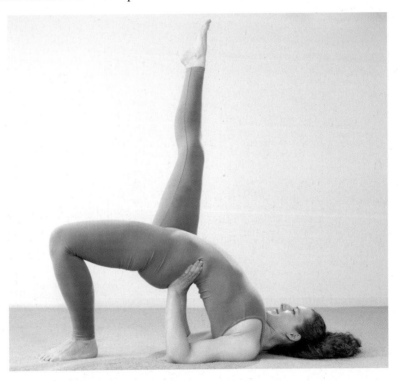

Gaze:	Center of the forehead.
Warm-ups:	Bridge Pose (page 64), Half Lotus (page 89), Single Leg Forward Bend (page 43).
Counterposes:	Wind Reliever (page 48), Reclined Hip Twist (page 22).
Easy variation:	Bridge Pose (page 64).
Benefits:	Strengthen and promotes flexibility for the spine; deep hip opener; prepares for the stronger hip stretches.
Breathing:	Exhale, press your back to the floor. Inhale, lift your spine into Bridge. Exhale, release spine to the floor.

FISH WITH LEGS AND ARMS EXTENDED

1. Begin lying on the mat, face up with your heels together, legs active, and buttocks tightened. Place your hands palms down with just your thumbs underneath your hips. Inhale and lift up through your chest to rest the crown of your head on the mat. Exhale, slide your thumbs out from underneath your hips. Activate your abdominal muscles.

2. Inhale and raise your legs and arms about forty-five degrees. Press your palms against each other. Breathe steadily.

3. Exhale and lower your arms and legs to the mat. Tuck in your chin to release your head to the floor.

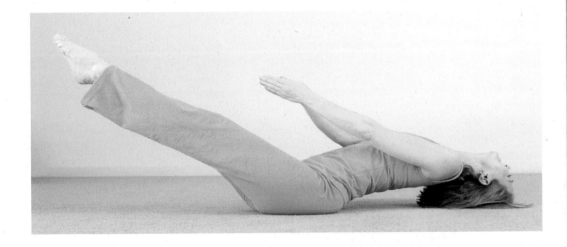

Gaze:	Center of the forehead.
Warm-ups:	Full Boat (page 51), Simple Fish (page 65), Bridge Pose (page 64).
Counterpose:	Wind Reliever (page 48).
Easy variation:	Simple Fish (page 65).
Benefits:	Increases strength and flexibility of the spine and lower back.
Breathing:	Inhale into pose, lifting your chest. Exhale, release your thumbs. Inhale, raise your arms and legs. Exhale to release out of the posture.

TWIST
WITH HANDS BEHIND THE BACK

1. Sit with your legs extended. Bend your left leg and bring your left heel to your left hip. Place your heel as close to your hip as possible.

2. Exhale, reach your left arm forward and around your left leg. Your right arm reaches around your right hip to catch hold of your left hand behind your back.

3. Inhale and extend through your spine, lift your heart, and open your right shoulder. Exhale, twist to the right. Breathe deeply in the posture. Release from the pose with an inhalation. Repeat on the other side.

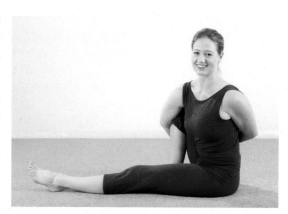

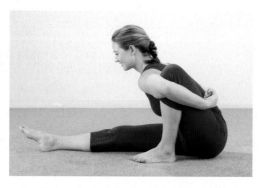

VARIATION WITH FORWARD BEND

4. To add the forward bend, from step 3, inhale and extend through your spine, lift your heart, and exhale into a forward bend. Bring your chest down toward your extended leg. Repeat on the other side.

Gaze:	Center of the forehead.
Warm-ups:	Half Twist II (page 156), Single Leg Forward Bend (page 43).
Counterpose:	Double Leg Forward Bend (page 42).
Easy variation:	Half Twist II (page 156).
Benefits:	Massages the internal organs; promotes a supple back and shoulders.
Breathing:	Inhale, lengthen your spine. Exhale, reach forward and around your back, catching hands. Inhale, lift your chest. Exhale, twist to look over your shoulder. Inhale, release the pose.

DOWNWARD FACING DOG WITH LEG EXTENDED

1. From Downward Facing Dog (page 73), shift your weight onto your right foot. Inhale, extend your left leg up as high as possible. Stretch through your toes. Keep your hips square to minimize any external rotation.

2. Exhale, release your right leg to the mat. Repeat on the other side.

3. As a variation, when one leg is extended, bend that leg and roll your hip up to the side.

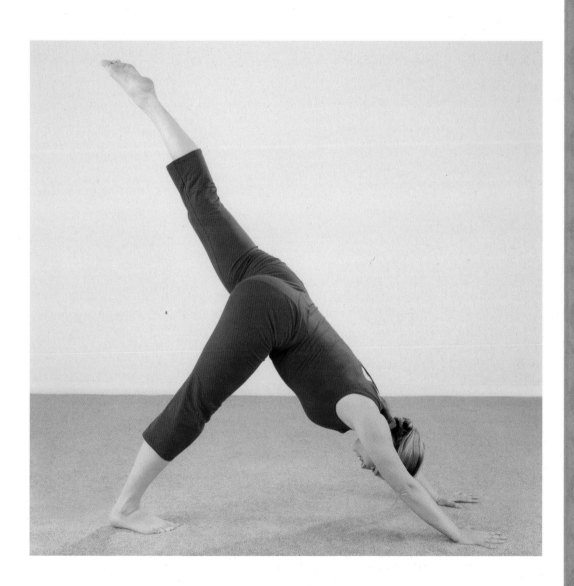

105

DOWNWARD FACING DOG WITH HALF LOTUS

1. Begin sitting with your legs crossed at one end of the yoga mat. Cradle your lower right leg to stretch your hip. Then place your ankle at the top of your left thigh in half lotus.

2. Inhale, lengthen your spine, and roll into a modified Table Pose (page 23). Curl your left toes under and exhale, lifting your hips into a modified Downward Facing Dog (page 73). Press down through your left heel. Activate your left thigh. Lift through your sit bones. Extend through your spine. Rotate your shoulder blades down and back toward your spine. Relax your head. Gaze at your knees.

3. Release from the pose by inhaling, dropping your knees into Table Pose (page 23), and exhaling into Half Lotus (page 89). Release the folded leg to the floor.

4. Repeat on the other side.

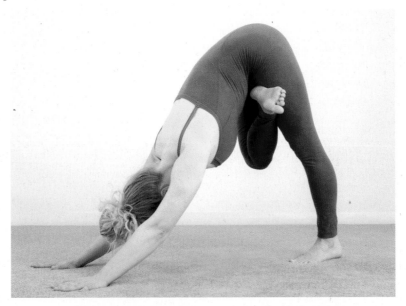

Gaze:	Gaze at the knees or the center of the forehead.
Warm-ups:	Half Lotus (page 89), Sitting Cradle Stretch (page 200), Downward Facing Dog (page 73), Lunges (page 22).
Counterposes:	Devotional Pose (page 207), Pigeon Pose with One Leg Extended (page 68), Crossbar (page 49).
Easy variation:	Downward Facing Dog (page 73).
Benefits:	Hip stretch to add the hamstring stretch.
Breathing:	Inhale, lengthen your spine and roll into Table. Exhale, press your hips up in Downward Facing Dog. Inhale back into Table. Exhale into Half Lotus.

SHOULDERSTAND TWIST

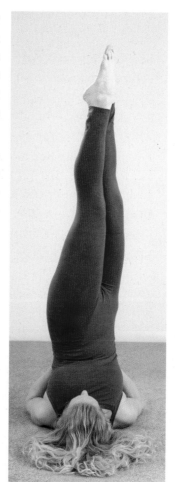

1. Begin lying on the yoga mat, face up. Prepare for Shoulderstand (page 70) by resting your shoulders on a folded blanket. Exhale and roll your knees up above your shoulders. Pause there to rotate your shoulders underneath your back. Interlace your fingers and bring your straight arms to the mat. Adjust your shoulders again, rotating them in further.

2. Release your hands and press them against your ribs to keep your torso vertical. Inhale and lift your legs into a vertical position over your shoulders. Pause here to adjust the pose. Press against your ribs to lift your torso straighter. Tuck in your pelvis. Activate your abdominal muscles and tone your legs. Point your toes and bring your feet over your eyes.

3. Exhale, twisting to the left by first rotating your torso, hips, and then your legs. Twist as far as possible to stretch your spine. Inhale to release back to center.

4. Switch sides. Exhale, twist to the right as far as possible. Inhale to come back to center.

5. Release from the pose by exhaling and lowering your legs. Release your hands to your sides. Inhale and roll out, returning to the floor.

Gaze:	Center of the forehead.
Warm-ups:	Bridge Pose (page 64), Simple Fish (page 65), Half Spinal Twist (page 52), Lunges (page 22).
Counterposes:	Simple Fish (page 65), Wind Reliever (page 48), Reclined Hip Rolls (page 54).
Easy variation:	Walk your feet up the wall and gently rotate to the left and to the right.
Benefits:	Massages the shoulders; stimulates the thyroid.
Breathing:	Exhale, roll your legs up above your shoulders. Inhale, lift your legs into the vertical position. Exhale, twist your legs and torso. Inhale, twist back to center. Exhale out of the pose.

SHOULDERSTAND WITH LEG EXTENDED

1. Begin lying on the yoga mat, face up. Prepare for Shoulderstand (page 70) by resting your shoulders on a folded blanket. Exhale and roll your hips up above your shoulders. Pause there to rotate your shoulders underneath your back. Interlace your fingers and bring your straight arms to the floor. Adjust your shoulders again, rotating them in further.

2. Release your clasped hands and press them against your ribs to keep your torso vertical. Inhale and lift your right leg so that your right knee is close to vertical over your shoulders. Pause here to adjust the pose. Press against your ribs to lift your torso straighter. Tuck in your pelvis. Activate your abdominal muscles and tone your legs. Press up through your extended leg.

3. Keeping your breath steady, work to deepen the pose. Use your torso muscles to lift and extend through your spine. Activate your abdominal muscles and your legs. Stretch up through your toes.

4. Release by exhaling and use your abdominal muscles to slowly lower your right leg down. Repeat once, extending your left leg up. Inhale, roll out across the mat to rest on your back. Exhale, relax.

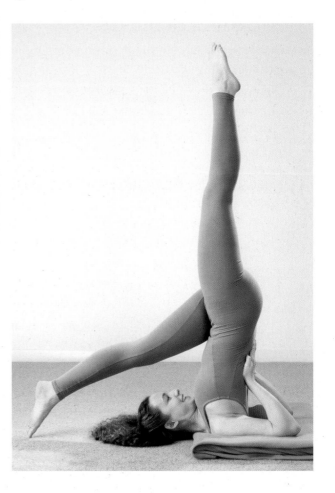

SHOULDERSTAND WITH HALF LOTUS

1. Begin lying on the mat, face up. Prepare for Shoulderstand (page 70) by resting your shoulders on a folded blanket. Fold your right leg into the half lotus posture. Exhale and roll your hips up above your shoulders. Pause there to rotate your shoulders underneath your back. Interlace your fingers and bring your straight arms to the floor. Adjust your shoulders again, rotating them in further.

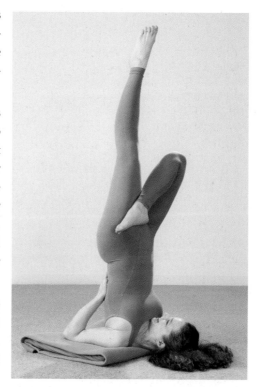

2. Release your clasped hands and press them against your ribs to keep your torso vertical. Inhale and lift your legs so that your right knee is close to vertical over your shoulders. Pause here to adjust the pose. Press against your ribs to lift your torso straighter. Tuck in your pelvis. Activate your abdominal muscles and tone your legs. Press up through your extended leg.

3. Keeping your breath steady, work to deepen the pose. Use your torso muscles to lift and extend through your spine. Activate your abdominal muscles and legs. Stretch up through your toes.

4. Release by exhaling and use your abdominal muscles to slowly lower your legs down, curling your knees toward your forehead. Inhale, roll out across the mat to rest on your back. Exhale, release the lotus posture. Repeat once, crossing your legs the other way.

Gaze:	Center of the forehead.
Warm-ups:	Full Lotus (page 90), Sitting Cradle Stretch (page 200), Lunges (page 22), Half Lotus (page 89), Cat-Cow (page 198), Bridge Pose (page 64), Shoulderstand (page 70).
Counterposes:	Simple Fish (page 65), Wind Reliever (page 48).
Easy variation:	Prop feet against the wall.
Benefits:	Strengthens the shoulders and back; opens the hips; massages the shoulders; stimulates the thyroid.
Breathing:	From the floor, exhale and roll your knees up above your shoulders, releasing your toes to the floor. Inhale and lift your legs up above your shoulders. Exhale to roll out of the pose.

PLOW TWIST

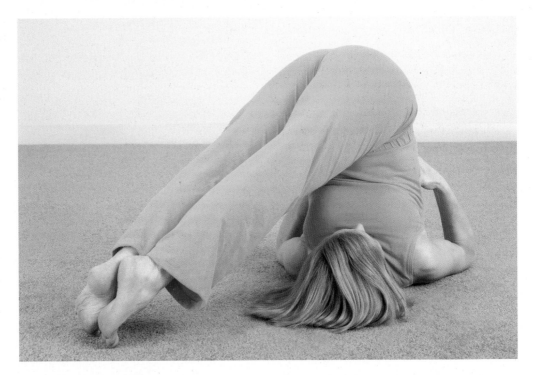

1. Begin doing the rollup for Shoulderstand (page 70). Exhale, bringing your toes all the way over your head to the mat. Exhale, twist to the left by walking your feet to the left. Twist as far as possible to stretch your spine. Inhale to twist and walk your feet back to center.

2. Switch sides. Exhale, twist to the right as far as possible.

3. Inhale to come back to center.

4. Release from the pose by exhaling and lowering your legs to the mat. Release your hands to your sides and inhale. Roll out, returning to the mat in Savasana (page 206).

Gaze:	Center of the forehead.
Warm-ups:	Bridge Pose (page 64), Shoulderstand (page 70), Simple Fish (page 65), Half Spinal Twist (page 52).
Counterposes:	Simple Fish (page 65), Wind Reliever (page 48), Half Spinal Twist (page 52).
Easy variation:	Walk feet up the wall and gently rotate to the left and to the right.
Benefits:	Massages the shoulders; stimulates the thyroid; stretches the spine and is a great warm up for Shoulderstand (page 70).
Breathing:	Exhale, roll your legs over your shoulders. On the next exhalation, begin rotating by walking your feet to one side. Inhale, rotate back to center. Exhale, roll your hips to the floor out of the pose. Inhale to lower your legs back to the mat in Savasana.

HEADSTAND TWIST

1. Begin in Headstand (page 72). To rotate in the pose, exhale, start from your torso and rotate your back, hips, and legs. Breathe fully and steadily. Inhale, release back to the center.

2. Exhale, rotate to the other side, beginning to twist through your spine, then hips, then legs. Inhale, rotate back to center.

3. Exhale and release from the pose. Lower your feet to the mat.

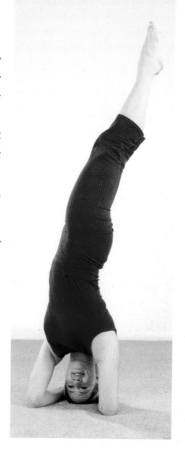

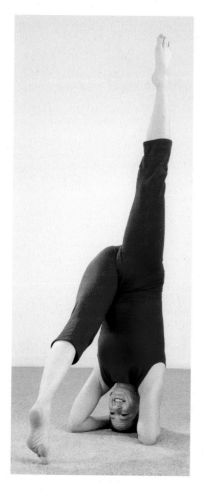

HEADSTAND WITH LEG EXTENSION

1. Prepare for the pose as in Headstand (page 72). Before kicking your legs up, shift your weight onto your right leg. Inhale and extend your left leg straight up. Keep your right leg strong and active. Exhale to release your left foot to the floor.

2. As an alternative, lift both legs straight and then lower one leg into the pose.

3. Repeat on the other side.

HEADSTAND SCISSOR LEG SPLIT TWIST

1. Begin in Headstand (page 72). Separate your feet as far as possible. Exhale and twist left, bringing your right leg in front and left leg behind. Move slowly and carefully in order to maintain balance.

2. Inhale, release back to center. Bring your ankles together. Exhale, repeat the twist on the other side.

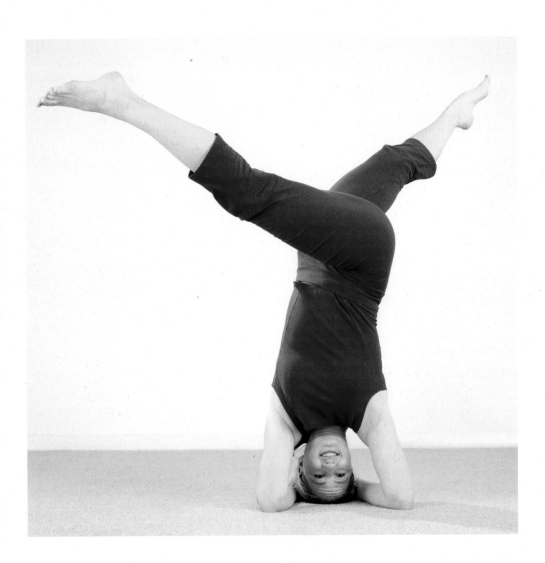

CROW HAND BALANCE

1. Begin in a squat position. Place your knees high up on your triceps. Exhale and tip forward, lifting one foot at a time. Bring your toes together while in the balance. Continue to breathe steadily.

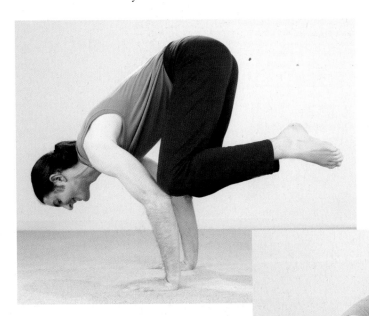

SIDE CROW HAND BALANCE

1. Begin in a squat and rotate strongly to the left. Rest your right knee on your left elbow. Exhale and tip forward, raising your hips. Your weight will primarily be on your left elbow. Turn your head to the left.

2. Exhale to release your feet down to the floor. Repeat on the other side.

Gaze:	Focus on a point between the eyebrows.
Warm-ups:	Half Lotus (page 89), Sitting Cradle Stretch (page 200), Downward Facing Dog (page 73), Lunges (page 22).
Counterposes:	Devotional Pose (page 207), Pigeon Pose with One Leg Extended (page 68), Crossbar (page 49).
Easy variation:	Downward Facing Dog (page 73).
Benefits:	Hip stretch to add the hamstring stretch.
Breathing:	Exhale, tip forward in the balance. Breathe in a steady manner. Exhale to release from the pose.

RESTING SIDE POSE

1. Begin lying on your right side. Raise your head about 45 degrees and support it with your right hand placed behind your ear. Inhale, draw your top arm and leg up to a 45 degree angle. Remain in the pose breathing naturally.

2. Exhale, release from the pose. Lower your top arm and leg. Repeat on the other side.

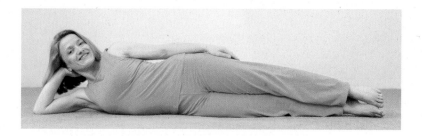

RESTING SIDE POSE II

1. Begin by lying on your right side. Extend your lower arm straight forward for balance. Inhale, bend your top leg and hook the first two fingers of your left hand around your big toe. Straighten your leg and raise it up as far as possible. Remain in the pose, breathing naturally.

2. Exhale, release from the pose. Lower your top arm and leg. Repeat on the other side.

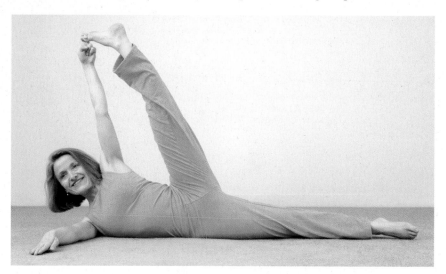

SIDE PLANK

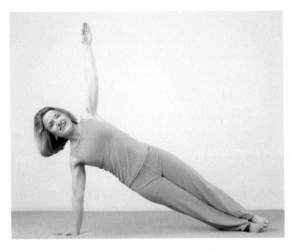

1. Begin in Plank Pose (page 200), positioning your hands under your shoulders like a push-up. Inhale and roll to the right. Position your right hand slightly in front of the line of your shoulder for easier balance. Extend your left arm straight up. Keep your legs stacked, ankles together, and press the soles of your feet toward the mat. Keep your legs, spine, and head aligned, and then breathe steadily.

2. Exhale out of the pose into Plank (page 200). Repeat on the other side.

SIDE PLANK WITH LEG EXTENDED

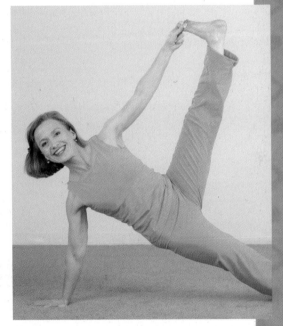

1. From Plank (page 200), inhale and roll into a Side Plank on your right side. Bend your left knee and reach down to grasp your big toe. With the next inhalation, draw your top foot up as high as possible. Balance here, breathing easily.

2. Exhale, release your foot and roll into Plank (page 200).

3. Repeat on the other side.

Gaze:	Center of the forehead.
Warm-ups:	Full Lotus (page 90), Sitting Cradle Stretch (page 200), Lunges (page 22), Half Lotus (page 89), Cat-Cow (page 198), Bridge Pose (page 64), Shoulderstand (page 70).
Counterposes:	Simple Fish (page 65), Wind Reliever (page 48).
Easy variation:	Use a yoga belt to support the raised leg.
Benefits:	Strengthens the shoulders and back; opens the hips; massages the shoulders; stimulates the thyroid.
Breathing:	Steady, even, full.

SIDE PLANK WITH HALF LOTUS

1. Begin sitting in Easy Sitting Pose (page 21). Cross your left leg into Half Lotus (page 89). Maintain Half Lotus and inhale, rolling forward into a modified Table Pose (page 23). Exhale and push into a modified Downward Facing Dog (page 73). Inhale and walk your hands forward to lower your hips into Plank (page 200). Roll into Side Plank (page 115), bringing your folded leg upward. Exhale to release out of the pose. Repeat on the other side.

2. For more challenge, this pose may be done with Bound Half Lotus. Begin sitting in Half Lotus with your left leg folded and resting on your right thigh. Reach your left arm behind your back to catch hold of your left foot. Support your weight on your right arm and straighten your body and legs. Lean onto your right hand and activate your entire body. Push up into the balance, maintaining the hold on your left foot. Exhale to release from the pose. Repeat on the other side. As an alternative, get into the pose using the method described in step 1, then drop your top arm down to catch your foot in Half Lotus (page 89).

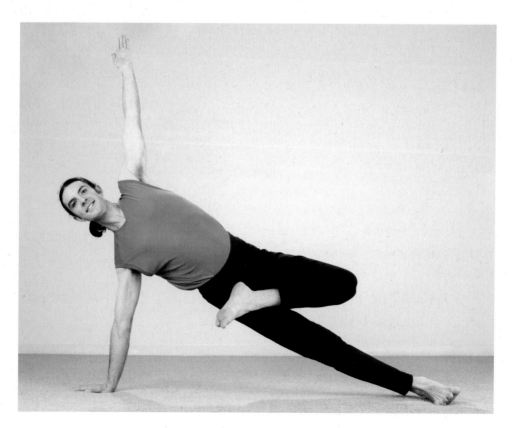

Home Practice Sequences

Nadi Sodhana

Nadi Sodhana restores balance to the flow of prana through the central nadis (subtle energy channels). The left nostril is the path of the Ida nadi, whose flow is cooling. The right nostril is the path of the Pingala nadi, whose flow is heating. Nadi Sodhana has the effect of calming the nerves and quieting the mind. If you are congested, practice a different style of breathing until the nostrils are clear again.

Use a simple hand position or mudra, where the second and third fingers are curled into the palm to regulate the alternate nostril breathing. The thumb and fourth fingers are placed where the nostrils flare and are used to direct breath flow by gently depressing the appropriate nostril. For right-handed people, raise the right hand and close the left nostril using the ring finger. Left-handed people may use the opposite hand and follow the instructions in reverse or from left side to right side.

Begin by breathing evenly. It calms the mind and brings an experience of balance and harmony. Each segment of the breath should be smooth and of equal length. It is very important to be relaxed, open, and unhurried when practicing this pranayama.

Candle Breath

This breathing style calms the emotions and quiets the mind. Breathe in deeply through the nose. Expand the abdomen and relax the shoulders and chest. Relax the jaw and the palate. Exhale in a soft, steady manner, rounding the mouth in an "O." Imagine that you are blowing out a candle in front of you. Repeat this practice three times, being aware of the calmness it creates.

Natural Breath Meditation

The ham sah mantra is considered the natural breath mantra. It is the sound the breath makes as it naturally flows in and flows out of the body. The mantra "ham sah" means "I am That." "That" refers to the consciousness that dwells within us as the Inner Self. Sit quietly and comfortably, and take a few moments to relax your body and mind. Notice your breath as you inhale and exhale. Don't try to alter or modify your breath; just observe it. As you relax during the inhalation, you will begin to hear the sound of ham as the breath enters your body. As you exhale, you will hear the sound of sah. The ham sah mantra is always present, whether you are aware of it or not. The process of meditation is to become consciously aware of this breath flow. The inhalation and exhalation are similar to a swinging pendulum. As the pendulum swings back and forth, there is a moment when all motion stops and the pendulum changes directions. Similarly, with the breath, between the inhalation and exhalation, the breath stops and changes directions. If you focus on the point of stillness between the ham and the sah, you will find that not only does the breath stop, but the mind stops as well. The breath and the mind are intertwined in this way.

This moment of silence, this moment where all mental, emotional, and physical activity ceases, is the gateway to the Inner Self. It is the experience of the pure consciousness that exists within you. As you sit in meditation, you might also notice that in between one thought and another thought there is the same instant when all activity stops. Focus your awareness on these still points between thoughts and between breaths. When you begin the practice, you might notice that your mind engages in some kind of activity: thinking about yesterday, or tomorrow's agenda, or some other distraction. When this happens, simply bring your attention back to the practice and don't worry about the distractions. When your mind becomes less agitated, you begin to experience pure consciousness, or the witness state. You begin to identify with the witness of all experience and activity. This witness is perfectly quiet, perfectly content, and dwells in perfect truth and bliss. This is an experience of your true nature.

Hatha Yoga Practice Sequence

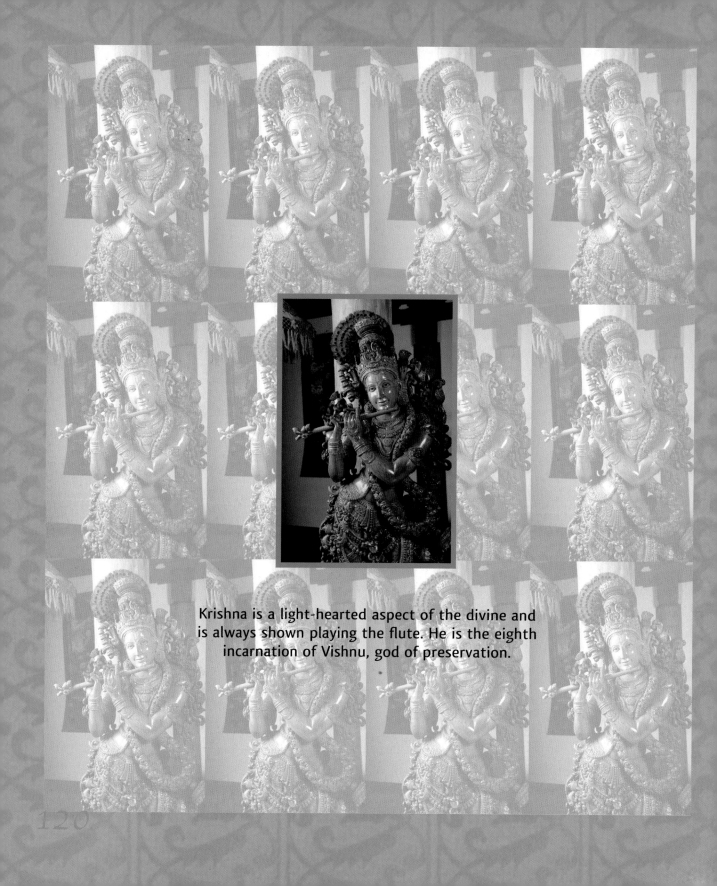

Krishna is a light-hearted aspect of the divine and is always shown playing the flute. He is the eighth incarnation of Vishnu, god of preservation.

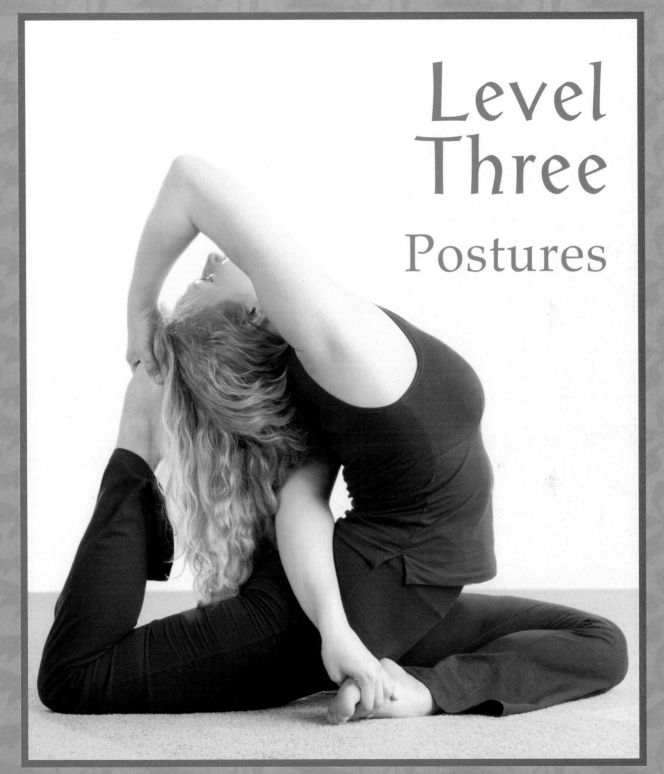

Level Three

Postures

Chapter Three

Level Three Postures

"Live fully, and love fully." – Faith Stone

CHAIR POSE

1. Stand in Mountain (page 26) at the end of the yoga mat. Exhale, bend your knees and fold into a Standing Forward Bend (page 37). Activate your thighs.

2. Inhale, sweep your arms out to the sides and up, lifting your chest and shoulders as much as possible. Bring your palms together with your arms resting at about 120 degrees from the floor. Gently gaze up to your hands. Breathe deeply, activating your thighs and toning the abdominal muscles.

3. Exhale, release your arms, and straighten your body back to Mountain (page 26).

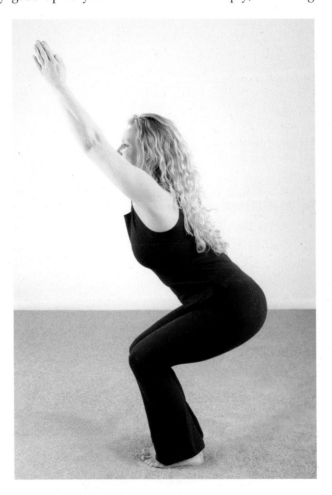

Gaze:	Look at hands.
Warm-ups:	Warrior I (page 27), Standing Head to Knee (page 39), Standing Head to Knee with Belt (page 41).
Counterposes:	Standing Forward Bend (page 37).
Easy variation:	Practice three in a row without holding the pose.
Benefits:	Strengthens the legs and back; invigorating.
Breathing:	Exhale into Standing Forward Bend (page 37). Inhale into Chair Pose. Exhale, drop your arms, and return to Mountain (page 26).

123

SIDE CHAIR

1. Stand in Mountain (page 26) at the end of the yoga mat. Exhale, bend your knees and fold into a Standing Forward Bend (page 37). Activate your thighs.

2. Inhale into Chair Pose (page 123), sweeping your arms out to the sides and up, lifting your chest and shoulders. Bring your palms together with your arms resting at about 120 degrees from the floor. Gently gaze up to your hands. Breathe deeply, activating your thighs and toning the abdominal muscles.

3. Exhale, rotate to the right, bringing your left elbow to the outside of your right thigh. Press your palms together and lift your heart to the line of your hands.

4. To come out of the pose, exhale and release your arms down. Inhale and lift back to Mountain (page 26).

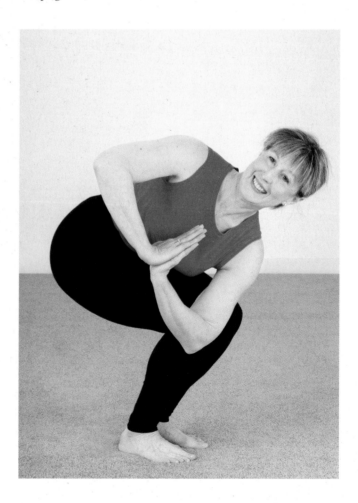

EAGLE

1. Stand in Mountain (page 26) at the end of the yoga mat. Establish steadiness in your breath. Shift your weight onto your right foot and slightly tuck in your pelvis. Bend your right leg and slowly twine your left leg around your right, hooking your foot behind your calf.

2. Inhale and stretch your arms to a T-position. Exhale and criss-cross your right arm over your left at the elbow. Intertwine your forearms. Bring your palms together.

3. To steady your balance, gaze at one point a body length away on the floor.

4. To release, exhale and return to Mountain (page 26).

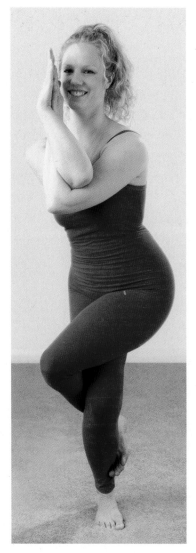

Gaze:	Center of the forehead.
Warm-ups:	Standing Forward Bend (page 37), Twisting Bear, (page 197), Sun Salutations (pages 76-79), Standing Head to Knee with Belt (page 41).
Counterposes:	Standing Forward Bend (page 37), Crescent Stretch (page 21).
Easy variation:	Cat-Cow (page 198).
Benefits:	Strengthens legs and back, and also promotes flexibility.
Breathing:	Use steady even breathing in Mountain (page 26). Twine your legs. Inhale, stretch your arms to T-position. Exhale, twine forearms and hands. Inhale, release from the pose into Mountain.

TIP TOE POSE

1. Stand in Mountain (page 26) at the end of the yoga mat. Bring your right foot to rest on the top of your left thigh in Half Lotus (page 89). If your foot slips, hold it in place.

2. Inhale, reach overhead to lengthen your spine. Exhale into a forward bend. The folded leg will remain in place now with your abdomen pressing into your left thigh.

3. Release your hands to the mat under your shoulders. Transfer your weight onto them and comfortably bend the support leg into a squatting position. Your right ankle will be resting on your left thigh.

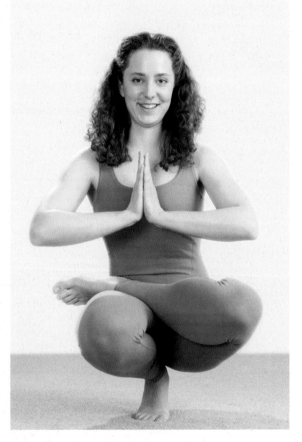

4. Bringing your palms together in front of your heart, balance on the ball of your left foot with your heel lifted. Your left center hamstring can rest on the calf muscle for support. If it's natural in the balance, your sit bone may rest on your heel.

5. To come out of the balance, exhale and place your hands under your shoulders. Lift your sit bones into a forward bend. Inhale to stretch your arms up, lifting your shoulder and head into a standing balance. Exhale to release your right leg down into Mountain (page 26).

6. As an alternative, begin this pose sitting in Half Lotus (page 89) and roll forward into the balance.

Gaze:	Center of the forehead.
Warm-ups:	Single Leg Forward Bend with Half Lotus (page 99), Sitting Cradle Stretch (page 200), Lunges (page 22).
Counterposes:	Shooting Star, Relaxing Forward Bend (page 200), Sitting Hip Rolls (page 199).
Easy variation:	Cross your ankles, but put both feet on the floor. Twine your forearms and hands, and exhale into a Forward Bend.
Benefits:	Strong hip opener; strengthens legs.
Breathing:	Inhale, stretch up with your free hand. Exhale, bend forward and lower into the balance. To release from the pose, exhale into Forward Bend. Inhale back to Mountain. Exhale to release the half lotus foot.

HORSE

1. Begin sitting in Half Lotus (page 89) with your right leg folded and resting on your left thigh. Inhale and roll forward, placing your hands on the mat. Step your left foot forward. Exhale and shift your weight slightly onto your right knee. Your left leg is forward in lunge position with your foot flat on the mat.

2. Inhale, lifting your shoulders. Draw up through your abdomen and tuck in your pelvis to adjust the balance.

3. Bring your palms together in front of your heart. Lift through your spine and the top of your head.

4. Exhale and release your hands back to the mat to come out of the pose. Roll back into a sitting position.

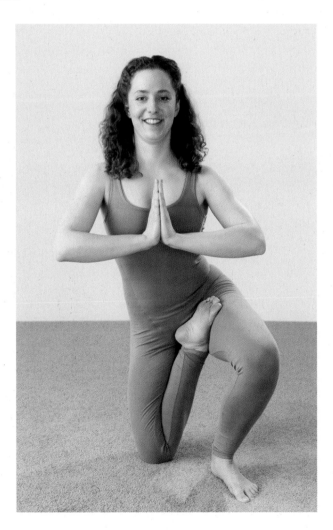

UPWARD BOW

1. Begin on your back on the yoga mat. Activate your abdominal muscles. Place both feet on the mat as close to your hips as possible. Place your hands in reverse beside your ears, fingertips reaching underneath your shoulders.

2. Exhale, press your lower back to the floor. Tone your buttocks and inhale, lifting your hips. Lift into the pose in two stages. Stage I: Arch and lift your back enough to rest the top of your head on the floor. Stage II: Taking another breath, exhale and extend fully into the backbend.

3. Once arched, shift your hands and feet by walking them closer together. Keep your feet parallel to each other. Extend fully through your spine. Draw your shoulder blades down and in toward your spine to fully open your shoulders. Lift through your rib cage.

4. Exhale, release from the pose, tucking your chin. Place the back of your head and shoulders on the mat and lower your spine. Stretch your legs out and relax your arms to the sides. Curl up in Double Leg Wind Reliever (page 48) to relax your back.

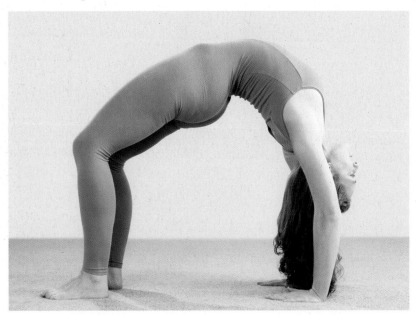

Gaze:	Center of the forehead.
Warm-ups:	Bridge Pose (page 64), Standing Head to Knee with Belt (page 41).
Counterpose:	Wind Reliever (page 48), Supine Cross-Legged Twist (page 205).
Easy variation:	Bridge Pose (page 64).
Benefits:	Exhilarating and energizing; opens the energy channels of the spine; strengthens and promotes flexibility of the legs, hips, spine, and shoulders.
Breathing:	Exhale, press your lower back to the floor. Inhale, press into the pose. Take two breaths to fully extend in the pose. Exhale to release.

UPWARD BOW WITH LEG EXTENSION

1. Begin on your back on the yoga mat. Activate your abdominal muscles. Place both feet on the mat as close to your hips as possible. Place your hands in reverse beside your ears, with your fingertips reaching underneath your shoulders.

2. Exhale, press your lower back to the floor. Tone your buttocks and inhale, lifting your hips. Lift into the pose in two stages: Stage I. Arch and lift your back enough to rest the top of your head on the floor; Stage II. Taking another breath, exhale and extend fully into the backbend.

3. Once arched, shift your hands and feet by walking them closer together. Step the left foot in towards the centerline of your body so it will be easier to balance. Inhale, bend your right knee, and draw it up above your hip, then straighten your leg with toes pointed. The extended leg will be almost perpendicular to the floor. Breathing steadily, extend fully through your spine.

4. Exhale, release the extended leg so that your foot returns to the mat. Release your spine. Switch sides and repeat.

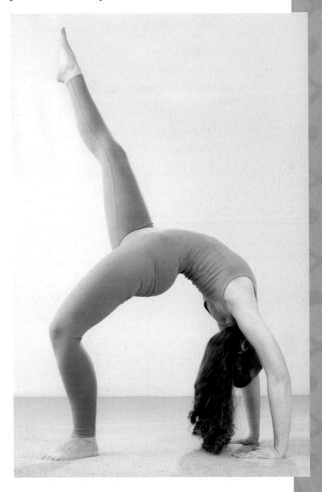

Urdhva Dhanurasana Eka Padasana

Gaze:	Center of the forehead.
Warm-ups:	Bridge Pose (page 64), Supine Leg Extensions (pages 203-204), Single Leg Forward Bend (page 43).
Counterposes:	Wind Reliever (page 48), Supine Cross-Legged Twist (page 205).
Easy variation:	Bridge Pose (page 64).
Benefits:	Strengthens and promotes flexibility for the spine; deep hip opener; prepares for stronger hip stretches.
Breathing:	Exhale, press your back to the floor. Inhale, lift your spine into Bridge. Exhale, release your spine to the floor.

CROWN PIGEON

1. Begin sitting with legs crossed. With hands on the mat shoulder distance apart, lean forward and place your right knee underneath your shoulders with your right foot under your left hip. Stretch your left leg straight back with your kneecap and the top of your foot on the floor. Extend in a back bend, resting your hands lightly on the floor beside your hips for balance. Breathe steadily and easily. Let your back muscles and hip flexors relax into the pose.

2. Bend the extended left leg so the ankle swings up above the knee. Inhale, extend through your spine, chest, and right shoulder. Reach your right hand back to catch your left foot. Reach your left hand back for the foot, as well. Remain in the posture, breathing fully and steadily.

3. Exhale to release from the pose, letting go of your foot and placing your hands on the sides of your hips. Relax your left leg to the floor.

4. Rest in Devotional Pose (page 207). Then switch sides.

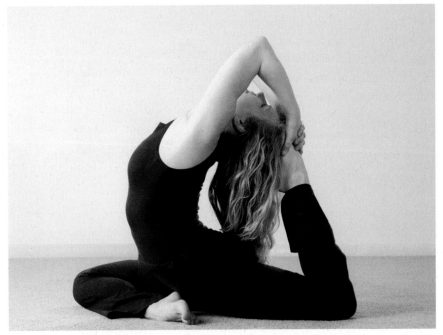

Gaze: Center of the forehead.
Warm-ups: Bridge Pose (page 64), Sitting Cradle Stretch (page 200), Half Lotus (page 89), Scissor Split (page 134), Upward Bow (page 128).
Counterpose: Devotional Pose (page 207).
Easy variation: Keep the back leg extended.
Benefits: Tremendous opening for the shoulders, hips, and spine.
Breathing: Inhale, extend your spine. Exhale, reach for your foot. Exhale, release from the pose.

SIDE CROWN PIGEON

1. Begin sitting with your legs crossed. With your hands on the floor shoulder distance apart, lean forward and place your right knee underneath your shoulders with your right foot under your left hip. Stretch your left leg straight back with your kneecap and the top of your foot on the floor. Extend in a back bend, resting your hands lightly on the floor beside your hips for balance. Breathe steadily and easily. Let your back muscles and hip flexors relax into the pose.

2. Bend the extended left leg so the ankle swings up above the knee. Inhale, extend through your spine, chest, and right shoulder. Exhale, reach your left arm back to catch your left foot. Reach to catch both hands above your head. Remain in the posture, breathing fully and steadily.

3. Exhale to release from the pose, letting go of your foot and placing your hands on the sides of your hips. Relax your left leg to the floor.

4. Rest in Devotional Pose (page 207). Then switch sides.

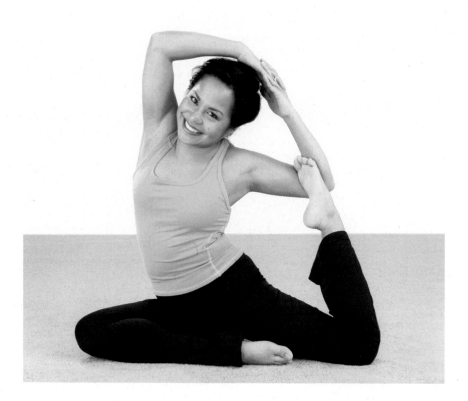

BOUND CROWN PIGEON

1. Begin sitting with your legs crossed. With your hands on the floor shoulder distance apart, lean forward and place your right knee underneath your shoulders with your right foot under your left hip. Stretch your left leg straight back with your kneecap and the top of your foot on the floor. Extend in a back bend, resting your hands lightly on the floor beside your hips for balance. Breathe steadily and easily. Let your back muscles and hip flexors relax into the pose.

2. Bend the extended left leg so the ankle swings up above the knee. Inhale, extend through your spine, chest, and right shoulder. Reach your left hand back to catch your left foot.

3. Reach your right hand around your lower back for your right foot. Remain in the posture, breathing fully and steadily.

4. Exhale to release from the pose, letting go of both feet. Place your hands on the sides of your hips. Relax your left leg to the floor.

5. Rest in Devotional Pose (page 207). Then switch sides.

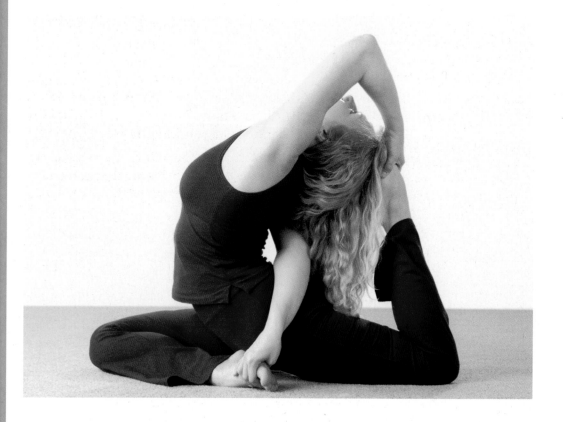

PIGEON

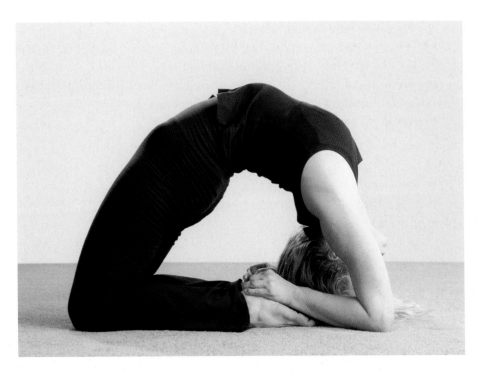

1. Begin in an upright kneeling position. Inhale and lengthen your spine. Exhale and lean back gently, reaching for your right heel with your right hand. Lean further, bringing your right elbow to the floor. Reach overhead, bringing your left elbow to the floor. Slide both hands underneath your shoulders, reaching for your feet.

2. Extend through your spine and press forward and up through your pelvis. Gently retract your shoulder blades. Remain in the pose, breathing steadily. To release, tuck your chin slightly in, exhale, and lower your spine to the floor. Inhale, release your arms to the side, and stretch your legs out.

Gaze:	Center of the forehead.
Warm-ups:	Bridge Pose (page 64), Camel (page 62), Upward Bow (page 128).
Counterpose:	Devotional Pose (page 207).
Easy variation:	Camel (page 62).
Benefits:	Tremendous opening for the shoulders, hips, and spine.
Breathing:	Inhale, extend your spine. Exhale, reach back. Inhale, lift your head, and exhale, release from the pose.

SCISSOR SPLIT

1. Begin kneeling. Extend your right leg forward in a lunge. Sink down into a strong groin stretch, and then fully extend your front leg with knee and toes up. Extend your back leg behind, bringing your knee to the floor and stretching out through your toes. Your hips should remain squared forward and your legs should remain active. Slightly tone your abdomen. There will be a light back extension.

2. Inhale and raise your arms over your shoulders, anchoring your shoulder blades. Lift through your heart.

3. Release from the pose by exhaling. Lower your arms and press your hands to the floor. Lift your hips slightly to bend your back leg. Move back into a sitting position.

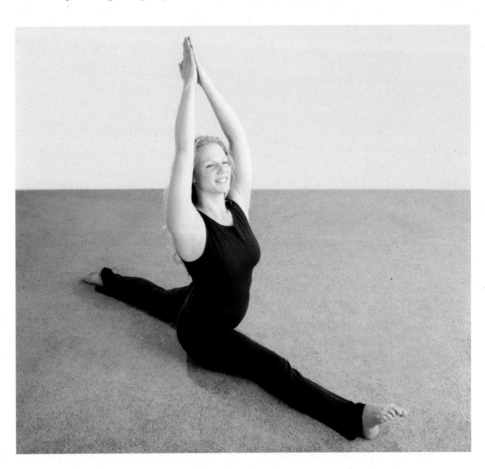

SHOULDERSTAND WITH LOTUS

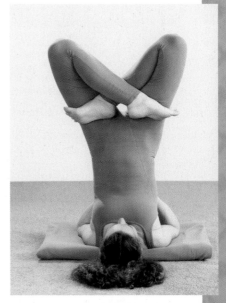

1. Begin in Full Lotus (page 90). Exhale, roll your legs back over your shoulders. Adjust your shoulders by bringing your shoulder blades in toward your spine.

2. Inhale, move your folded legs into a vertical posture by pressing up through both knees. Tuck in your pelvis to lengthen your spine.

3. Exhale, roll out of the pose gently, curling your legs for comfort. Repeat the posture with your legs crossed in the reverse.

4. Practice Simple Fish (page 65) and Wind Reliever (page 48) after shoulderstands.

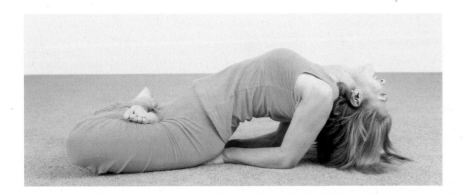

FISH WITH LOTUS

1. Begin in Full Lotus (page 90). Position your hands palms down with your fingertips underneath your hips.

2. Exhale, lean onto your elbows, dropping your head back. Position your elbows underneath your ribs. Draw your shoulder blades in toward your spine for support. Lift through your heart.

3. Inhale, lift your head to begin coming out of the pose. Press down through your palms and straighten your arms, lifting back to a sitting posture.

4. Exhale, release your hands and legs. Repeat the posture with your legs crossed in the reverse.

SHOULDERSTAND WITH SIDE LOTUS

1. Begin in Full Lotus (page 90). Exhale, roll your legs back over your shoulders. Adjust your shoulders by bringing your shoulder blades in toward your spine.

2. Inhale, move your folded legs into a vertical posture by pressing up through both knees. Tuck in your pelvis to lengthen your spine.

3. Exhale, continue to arch your back, placing your left hand underneath your left gluteal muscles. Press your right hand against your right ribs for support.

4. Lower your legs into a gentle back extension. Maintain balance with steady breathing and concentration.

5. Inhale, lift your legs back to center to switch sides. Change hand positions and swivel to the opposite side.

6. Exhale, lower your legs into a gentle back extension. Maintain balance. Inhale, lift your legs back to center.

7. Exhale, roll out of the pose gently, curling your legs forward for comfort. Repeat the posture with your legs crossed in the reverse.

8. Practice Simple Fish (page 65) and Wind Reliever (page 48) poses after shoulderstands.

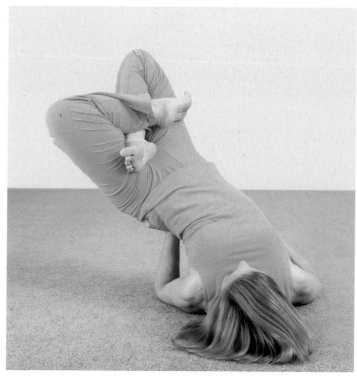

KNEE TO EAR POSE

1. Begin sitting with your legs crossed. Exhale, recline, and roll both legs over your shoulders into Plow (page 71). Pause to draw your shoulder blades in toward your spine. Press both hands against your back ribs.

2. Exhale, lower your knees to the floor beside your ears. Relax your breath in order to accommodate the tight curl on the torso. Breathe deeply.

3. Inhale, release out of the pose by lowering your back to the floor. Exhale, release your legs to the floor.

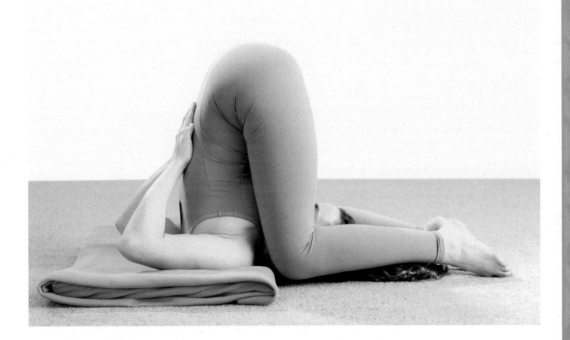

Gaze:	Center of the forehead.
Warm-ups:	Plow (page 71), Shoulderstand (page 70), Double Leg Forward Bend (page 42).
Counterposes:	Simple Fish (page 65), Shoulderstand (page 70), Wind Reliever (page 48), Reclined Hip Rolls (page 54).
Benefits:	Massages internal organs; strong shoulder and neck stretch.
Breathing:	Exhale, roll into Plow and lower your knees to your ears. Inhale, come out of the pose and release your back to the floor. Exhale, release your legs to the floor.

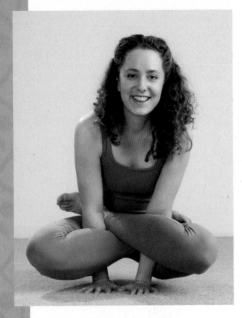

ROOSTER

1. Begin in Full Lotus (page 90). Slide your right arm through the fold at your right knee up to your forearm. Slide your left arm through the fold at your left knee up to your forearm.

2. Position your hands on the floor, palms down with your fingers evenly spread. Inhale, lift your knees to activate the abdominal muscles. Exhale, press into the pose.

3. Exhale, release from the pose, and undo your arms and legs. Repeat with your legs crossed in Full Lotus so the opposite leg is on top.

EMBRYO

1. Begin in Full Lotus (page 90). Slide your right arm through the fold at your right knee up to your forearm. Slide your left arm through the fold at your left knee up to your forearm.

2. Position your hands on the floor palms down, with your fingers evenly spread. Inhale, lift your knees to activate your abdominal muscles. Exhale, push down through your hands to roll back into a balance. Distribute your weight as if in Full Boat (page 51), balancing between your sit bones and the back of your hips.

3. Exhale, release from the pose, and undo your arms and legs. Repeat with your legs crossed in Full Lotus so the opposite leg is on top.

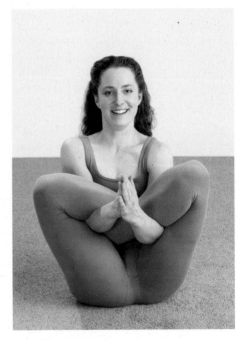

Gaze:	Center of the forehead.
Warm-ups:	Full Boat (page 51), Sitting Cradle Stretch (page 200), Double Leg Forward Bend (page 42).
Counterposes:	Sitting Hip Rolls (page 199), Wind Reliever (page 48), Reclined Hip Twist (page 22).
Benefits:	Massages internal organs; strong shoulder and neck stretch.
Breathing:	Inhale, lift your knees. Exhale, push into the balance. Come out of the pose, exhale, and release your legs to the floor.

ARM BALANCE WITH LEG EXTENSION

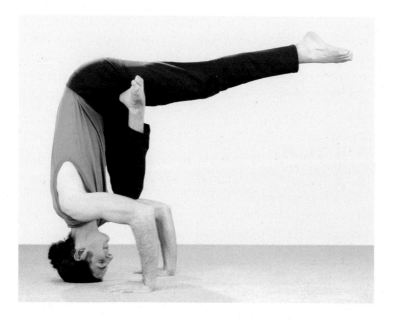

1. Begin sitting in Half Lotus (page 89). Inhale and roll forward in order to place your head on the floor.

2. Place the half lotus leg on your elbow, and stretch your other leg out behind and parallel to the floor.

3. Inhale, lift your head and shoulders, and balance on both hands.

4. Exhale, release out of the pose. Repeat on the other side.

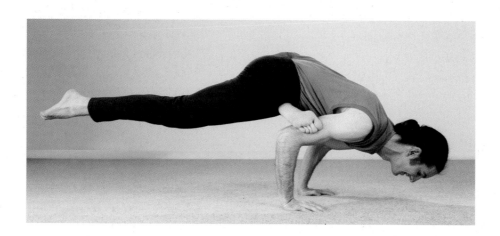

SHOULDERSTAND WITH ARMS TO FLOOR BEHIND

1. Begin lying on the floor, face up. Prepare for Shoulderstand (page 70), by resting your shoulders on a folded blanket. Exhale and roll your knees up above your shoulders. Pause there to rotate your shoulders underneath your back. Interlace your fingers and bring your straight arms to the floor. Again adjust your shoulders, rotating them in further.

2. Release your hands and press them against your back ribs to keep your torso vertical. Inhale and lift your legs into a vertical position over your shoulders. Press against your back ribs to lift your torso straighter. Tuck in your pelvis. Activate your abdominal muscles and tighten your legs. Point your toes and bring your feet over your eyes.

3. Keeping your breath steady, gently lower your arms to the floor behind your back. Use your torso muscles to lift and extend through your spine. Activate your abdominal muscles and legs. Stretch up through your toes.

4. Release by exhaling and, using your abdominal muscles, slowly lower your legs into Plow (page 71). Inhale and roll out across the floor to rest on your back.

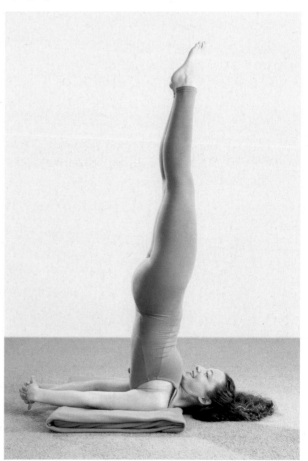

SHOULDERSTAND WITH ARMS TO FLOOR OVERHEAD

1. Begin lying on the floor, face up. Prepare for Shoulderstand (page 70), by resting your shoulders on a folded blanket. Exhale and roll your knees up above your shoulders. Pause there to rotate your shoulders underneath your back. Interlace your fingers and bring your straight arms to the floor. Adjust your shoulders again, rotating them in further.

2. Release your hands and press them against your back ribs to keep your torso vertical. Inhale and lift your legs into a vertical position over your shoulders. Press against your back ribs to lift your torso straighter. Tuck in your pelvis. Activate your abdominal muscles and tone your legs. Point your toes and bring your feet over your eyes.

3. Keeping the breath steady, gently lower your arms to the floor behind your head. Use your torso muscles to lift and extend through your spine. Activate your abdominal muscles and your legs. Stretch up through your toes.

4. Release by exhaling and, using your abdominal muscles, slowly lower your legs into Plow (page 71). Inhale and roll out across the floor to rest on your back.

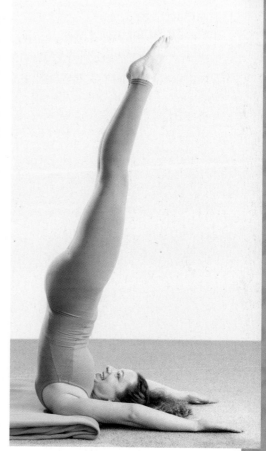

Gaze:	Center of the forehead.
Warm-ups:	Bridge Pose (page 64), Simple Fish (page 65), Shoulderstand (page 70).
Counterposes:	Simple Fish (page 65), Wind Reliever (page 48).
Easy variation:	Prop your feet against the wall.
Benefits:	Strengthens the shoulders and back, massages the shoulders, stimulates the thyroid.
Breathing:	From the floor, exhale and roll your knees up above your shoulders, releasing your toes to the floor. Inhale and lift your legs up above your shoulders. Exhale, release back to the floor.

SHOULDERSTAND WITH ARMS STRAIGHT UP

1. Lift up into Shoulderstand with Arms to Floor Behind (page 140). Inhale and gently raise your arms toward your hips, right next to your body. Use your torso muscles to lift and extend through your spine. Activate your abdominal muscles and your legs. Stretch up through your toes.

2. Release by exhaling and, using your abdominal muscles, slowly lower your legs into Plow (page 71). Inhale and roll out across the floor to rest on your back.

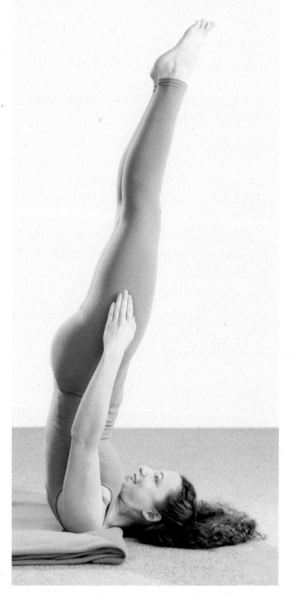

Gaze:	Center of the forehead.
Warm-ups:	Bridge Pose (page 64), Simple Fish (page 65), Shoulderstand (page 70).
Counterposes:	Simple Fish (page 65), Wind Reliever (page 48).
Easy variation:	Prop your feet against the wall.
Benefits:	Strengthens the shoulders and back, massages the shoulders, stimulates the thyroid.

FOREARM BALANCE

1. Begin in Devotional Pose (page 207). Stretch your arms out across the floor, shoulder distance apart. Keep your elbows shoulder distance apart. Activate your arms and shoulders.

2. Pressing on your forearms, exhale to kick your legs up. A gentle curve throughout your spine is normal. Tone your torso, buttocks, and legs. Keep your heels together. Position your head so that your face is toward the floor. Your shoulder joints will be over your elbows. Gently gaze at the point between your eyebrows.

3. Exhale, release from the pose, and lower your feet to the floor. Stay in Devotional Pose (page 207) for a few breaths.

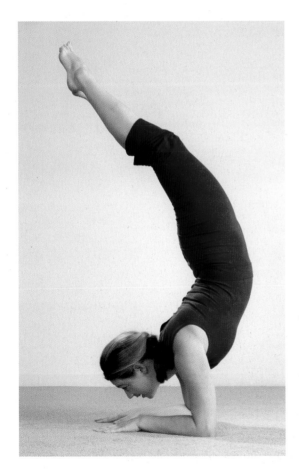

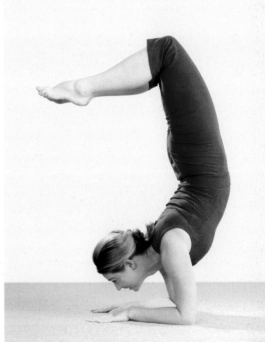

**Forearm Balance
with Slight Curl**

143

HANDSTAND

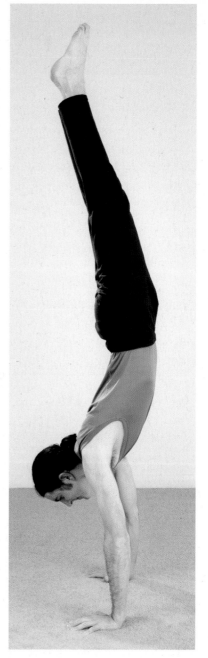

1. Begin with your hands on the floor a little wider than shoulder distance apart. To start, kick up against a wall. When you are steadier in this balance, kick up in the middle of the room. Activate your arms and anchor your shoulders for support.

2. Inhale and lift your legs above your hips and shoulders. Strengthen and tone your entire body. Extend through your toes. Your back may arch a bit to help balance. Breathe steadily.

3. Exhale to release from the pose, lowering your legs. Pause for a time in Devotional Pose (page 207) to let the circulation return to normal.

Gaze:	Center of the forehead.
Warm-ups:	Downward Facing Dog (page 73), Lunges (page 22), Shoulderstand (page 70), Headstand (page 72).
Counterposes:	Devotional Pose (page 207), Cat-Cow (page 198), hand stretches.
Easy variation:	Turn your back to a wall and from Standing Forward Bend (page 37), walk your feet up the wall.
Benefits:	Circulation is reversed and increased to the upper extremities.
Breathing:	Inhale, extend your legs up the wall. Exhale, lower your legs.

POSE OF REPOSE OR ELBOW DANCE

1. Begin in Devotional Pose. As you start learning the pose, place your fingertips six to ten inches from the bottom of a wall and kick up against the wall. Later, when your balance is steadier, kick up in the middle of the room. A quiet inner focus helps you stay balanced in the pose.

2. To position your arms, first stretch them out across the floor shoulder distance apart. Then bend your arms and rest your chin in your palms. Curl your fingers out to the sides of your cheeks.

3. Activate your arms, shoulders, and abdominal muscles. Press down on your elbows and exhale to lift your hips. Find balance on your elbows and toes. Concentrate.

4. Exhale, kick up into the elbow balance. Straighten your legs. A gentle curve throughout your spine is normal. Tone your abdominal muscles, buttocks, and legs. Keep your ankles together. Gently gaze at the point between your eyebrows. Continue to breathe steadily.

5. Exhale, release from the pose, and lower your feet to the floor. Stay in Devotional Pose (page 207) for a few breaths.

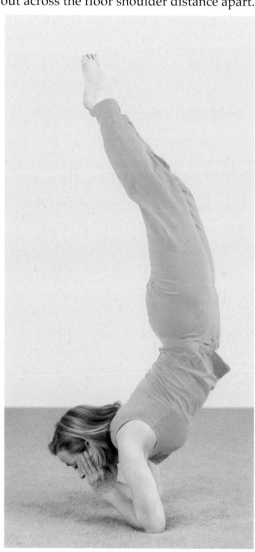

145

Home Practices

Basic Tension Release Practice

Begin by taking a deep breath into your heart, and feel it open and expand. On the next breath, imagine the energy of the breath (called prana) flow between your brows and down through your throat. Swallow to relax your throat, dropping the energy down into your heart center. Now hold the breath in your heart area. As you hold the breath in your heart, silently repeat "I wish to release all negative psychic tension." Feel the pure energy of the breath begin to break up blockages or tensions anywhere in you. Then, on the exhalation, your arms become like conduits for releasing this negative psychic energy. Imagine that these tensions become a smoky, dark liquid that easily flows down your arms, through your hands, and disappears through the floor.

Continue this process for as long as you would like. The key to this practice is deeply asking to let go of these negative psychic tensions and allowing the pure prana of the breath to fill you. There is no need to analyze what is being released. Just allow these old patterns to disappear and open to receive a much higher energy with each breath.

Heart Meditation

This meditation practice involves bringing your focus to the energy center located in the middle of your chest, next to the physical heart. This center is called anahata chakra, and it can serve as a powerful entryway to higher realms of awareness. The spiritual heart is the seat of consciousness. To begin the practice, watch your breathing without any judgment. Notice each time you inhale and exhale. Pay special attention to your heart area; as you inhale, expand in this area as much as you can. Allow the breath to be natural, not forced. It isn't necessary to take very deep breaths in order to focus on your heart. Visualize and feel your heart opening like a flower opening. This expansion is not bound by the limits of the physical body, but can continue endlessly. As you exhale, relax in the heart area. Notice any feelings of peacefulness and quiet. Each time you inhale, feel expansion. Each time you exhale, feel the peace and relaxation. As you watch your breathing, begin to release all thoughts, emotions, and mental activity. Feel them dissolve and melt away. Continue to follow your breath into your heart. Bring the sense of self that you carry in your mind down to your heart by shifting attention from your mind to your heart. Breathe into your heart center, let go of your desire, definition, and philosophy, and simply feel your heart center expand. Hold your attention in your heart as you slowly release your breath. As the stresses of everyday life swirl around you, it is helpful to take time to center yourself in your heart. When you do this practice, you will begin to experience the nature of your heart center. As you become more and more aware of your spiritual heart, it will become easier for you to let go of your thoughts, emotions, and obscurations. You will begin to experience a state of peace and clarity that you can carry with you in all situations or circumstances.

Hatha Yoga Practice Sequence

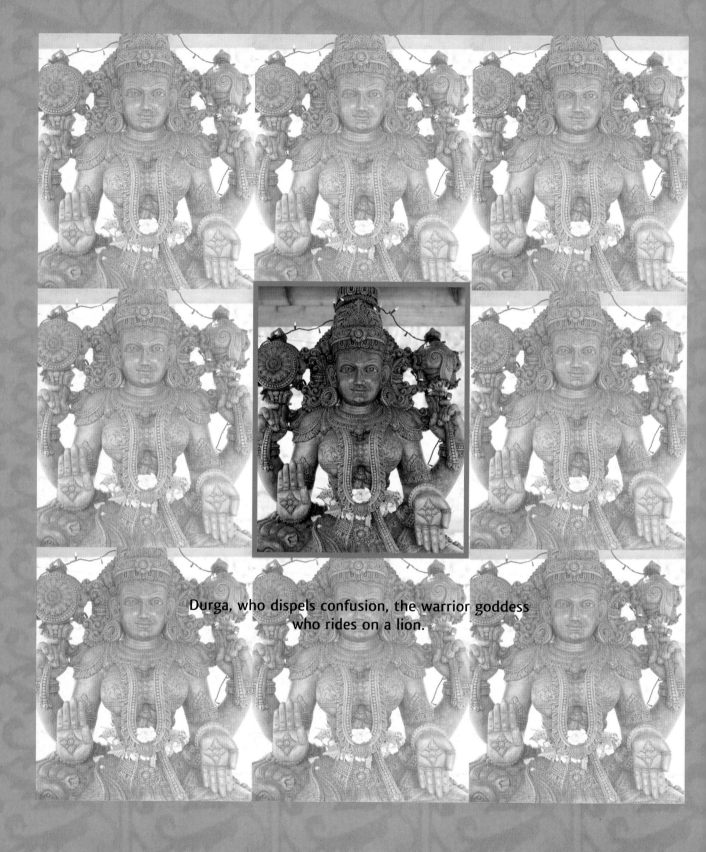

Durga, who dispels confusion, the warrior goddess
who rides on a lion.

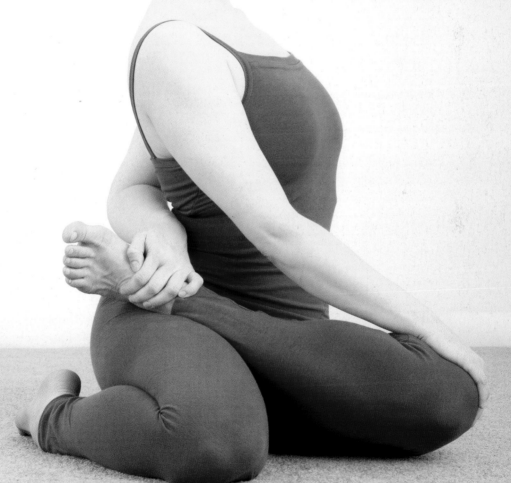

Level Four

Postures

Chapter Four

Level Four Postures

"Love is the greatest gift that we have to give as human beings."
– Faith Stone

UPWARD FACING DOUBLE LEG FORWARD BEND I

1. Begin in Staff Pose (page 23) with both legs extended forward. Balance as in Full Boat (page 51). Lean back to engage your abdominal muscles. Draw your legs up with your knees bent so your lower legs will be parallel to the floor.

2. Reach for your heels or toes and exhale, extending your legs forward and up. Keep your abdominal muscles tightened. Keep your back straight and lift through your chest.

3. Balance in the posture, breathing steadily and easily. Maintain a calm inner focus. As comfort increases, draw your legs in closer to your torso.

4. Exhale, release from the pose. Bend your knees, let go of your feet, and bring your toes to the floor.

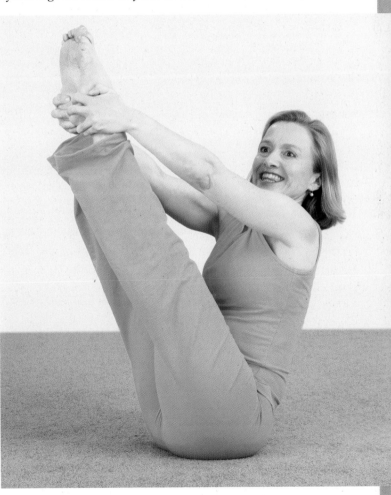

UPWARD FACING DOUBLE LEG FORWARD BEND II

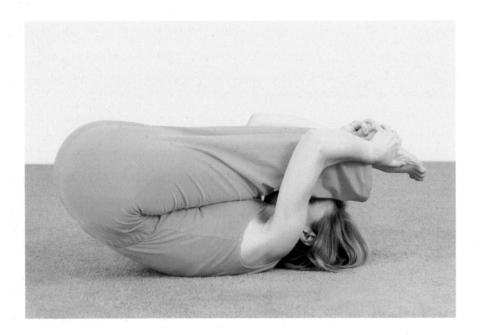

1. Begin lying on the floor, face up. Tone your legs and abdominal muscles. Keeping your back on the floor, exhale and extend your legs up above your hips and torso. Keeping your legs straight, reach for your heels.

2. Slowly draw your legs toward your torso, elbows out to the sides and chin resting below your knees. Your hips may lift up above the floor slightly, but your ribs and shoulders will remain down.

3. Breathe steadily and evenly while in the pose. Release from it by exhaling and lowering your feet to the floor.

Gaze:	Toes or center of the forehead.
Warm-ups:	Single Leg Forward Bend (page 43), Double Leg Forward Bend (page 42), Full Boat (page 51).
Counterposes:	Relaxing Forward Bend (page 200), Half Spinal Twist (page 52), Wind Reliever (page 48).
Easy variation:	Legs against wall, bent legs.
Benefits:	Good for the back and tones abdominal muscles.
Breathing:	Exhale, raise your legs and draw toward your torso. Steadily breathe in the pose. Exhale, release your legs to the floor.

HERON

1. Begin kneeling with your heels to the outside of your hips. Draw your right knee up toward your chest and reach both hands around your right heel. Exhale, lean back slightly and extend your right leg up. Keep your leg as straight as possible.

2. As comfort increases, draw the elevated leg closer into your torso, bringing your elbows out to the sides. Your upper back may round a little. Breathe steadily and work in the pose.

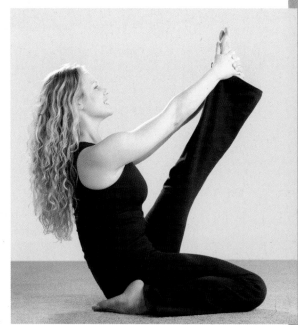

Gaze:	Toe or center of the forehead.
Warm-ups:	Single Leg Forward Bend (page 43), Half Spinal Twist (page 52).
Counterposes:	Sitting Child's Pose (page 22), Reclined Hip Twist (page 22).
Easy variation:	Curl your right leg in front like Single Leg Forward Bend (page 43); extend your left leg.
Benefits:	Increases flexibility in legs and hips, tones abdominal muscles.
Breathing:	Exhale, extend your leg. Exhale, release the pose.

HERON WITH HALF LOTUS

1. Begin sitting with your left leg in Half Lotus (page 89). Bend your right leg. Catch your hands behind your heel and lean back. Find a balance point, exhale, and extend your right leg. Keep your arms straight and tone your abdominal muscles. Balance with a steady even breath.

2. To release from the pose, exhale and bend your right leg. Release your foot to the floor. Relax your left leg out across the floor. Lean back to rest before working on the other side.

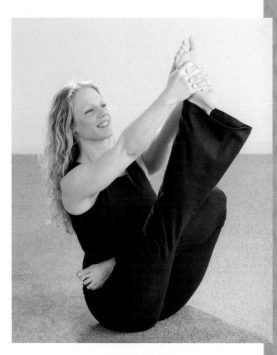

153

STANDING FORWARD BEND WITH LEG EXTENSION

1. Begin in Mountain (page 26). Exhale into Standing Forward Bend (page 37). Allow your right hand to grasp your right heel. Place your left hand on the floor.

2. Inhale, extending your left leg up as high as possible without rotating your hip. Activate both legs and point the toes on your left foot.

3. Exhale and lower your left foot to the floor.

4. Repeat on the other side.

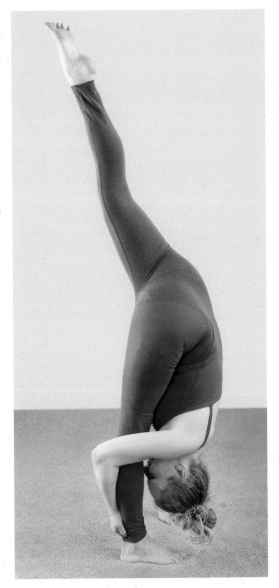

Gaze:	Center of the forehead.
Warm-ups:	Double Leg Forward Bend (page 42), Single Leg Forward Bend (page 43), Runner's Lunge (Step 4 in Sun Salutation, page 76), Scissor Split (page 134), Chair (page 123).
Counterposes:	Twisting Bear (page 197), Standing Forward Bend (page 37).
Benefits:	Greatly stretches hamstrings and hips.
Breathing:	Exhale into the Forward Bend. Inhale, raise one leg. Exhale and release.

LATERAL ANGLE WITH LEG EXTENSION

1. From Lateral Angle (page 29), take your lower arm underneath your front leg and your top arm around your back to grasp your fingers. Carefully shift your balance onto your front foot.

2. Inhale and raise your back leg, opening your hip forward and rotating through your ribs.

3. Exhale and release your top leg down. Release your hands.

4. Inhale back up to standing and exhale into Mountain (page 26). Repeat on the other side.

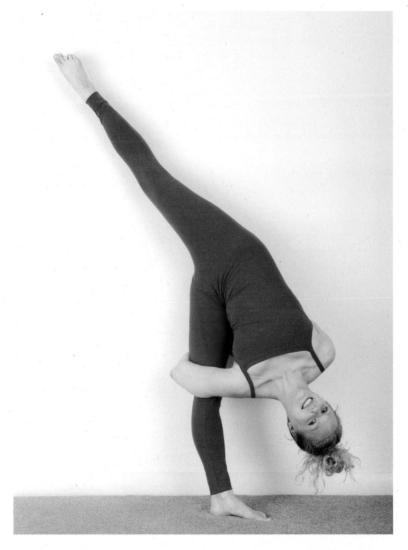

HALF TWIST II

1. Begin sitting with your legs stretched out. Fold your right leg into Half Lotus (page 89), resting your right foot on your left thigh.

2. Inhale, lengthen your spine. Exhale, rotate to the left with your left arm reaching behind your back to grasp your right ankle. Your right hand should reach for the outside edge of your left foot. Lift through your heart and open your left shoulder into the twist.

3. Inhale, release from the pose. Exhale, stretch both legs out and relax your hands to either side. Repeat on the other side.

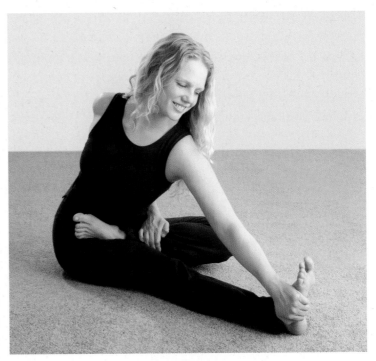

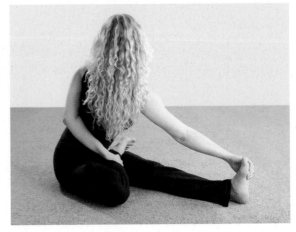

Gaze:	Big toe on extended leg.
Warm-ups:	Half Spinal Twist (page 52), Single Leg Forward Bend (page 43).
Counterposes:	Double Leg Forward Bend (page 42), Child's Pose (page 207).
Easy variation:	Single Leg Forward Bend with twist to folded knee.
Benefits:	Excellent twist for the spine and massage for the internal organs. Relieves stiffness in the lower back and hip joints.

TWIST WITH HALF LOTUS

1. Begin with your right foot resting on your left thigh in Half Lotus (page 89). Bend your left leg to place your left foot on the floor.

2. Reach your left arm around your left knee while reaching your right arm around your lower back. Catch your hands behind your back.

3. Lift your chest and exhale, rotating to the right. Draw your right shoulder blade toward your spine.

4. Inhale, rotate back to center. Exhale, release your arms and leg. Repeat on the other side.

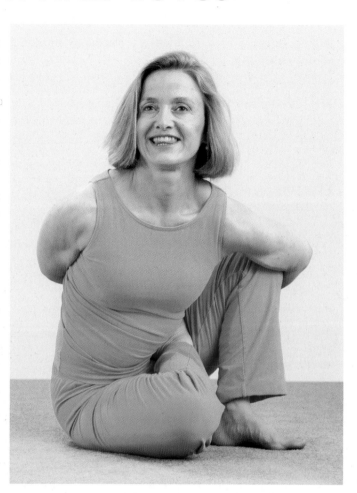

FROG

1. Begin lying face down on the floor. Rest your chin on the floor. Draw your ankles up above your knees.

2. Lift your torso up as in Cobra (page 56) and slide your left forearm under your shoulders for support. Reach your right hand back to your right foot. Open your right shoulder and roll your ribs to the right in order to reverse your right hand over the top of your foot. Your fingertips can then curl over your toes.

3. Repeat on the left.

4. With your hands on your feet and your full torso on the floor, inhale and press down on your feet, bringing your heels closer to the floor outside your hips. While pressing your feet simultaneously, lift your shoulders and head, and bend your elbows. Keep your knees on the floor. Your back extends gently.

5. Exhale and release from the pose, lowering your shoulders and arms. Release your feet and return your legs to the floor. Turn your head to one side to rest and absorb.

6. Press back into Devotional Pose (page 207) to relax your lower back.

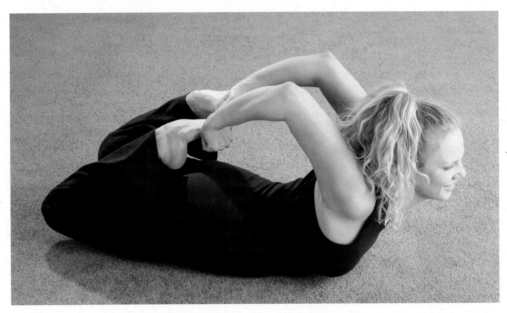

Gaze:	Center of the forehead.
Warm-ups:	Supine Hero (page 66), Cobra (page 56), Locust (page 59), Standing Head to Knee with Belt (page 41).
Counterpose:	Devotional Pose (page 207).
Easy variation:	Practice only one side at a time.
Benefits:	Increases circulation to the knees, ankles, and lower back.
Breathing:	Inhale, lift your shoulders and press down on your feet. Exhale to release out of the pose and rest on the floor.

LEAPING CROCODILE (PREP)

1. Begin in Table Pose (page 23). Position your hands underneath your shoulders. Tone your abdominal muscles. Step your feet back into Plank Pose (page 200), toning your legs, buttocks, and abdomen. Keep your heels together.

2. Exhale, lower your shoulders to about two inches above the floor. Remain in the pose with steady breathing.

3. Exhale, push back into Devotional Pose (page 207) to release from the pose.

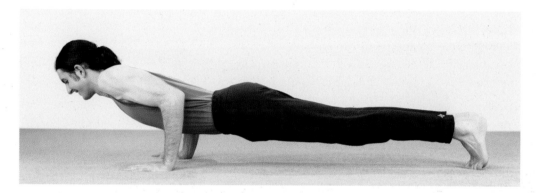

LEAPING CROCODILE

1. Begin lying face down. Bring your palms down underneath your shoulders. Curl your toes underneath your heels.

2. Inhale and lift into Chaturanga (page 201), then spring up into the air. Lift completely off the floor, pouncing forward one foot.

3. Land on your hands and feet just as you started. Repeat twice more. Also try pouncing in reverse.

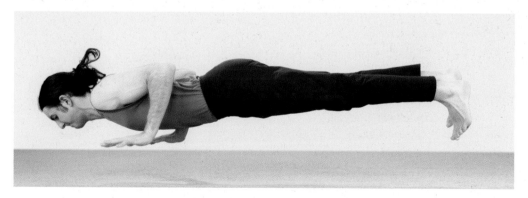

PEACOCK

1. Begin in Table Pose (page 23) with your hands underneath your ribs. Place your palms down with your fingertips toward your toes. Position your elbows in your solar plexus.

2. Strongly activate your abdominal muscles and lean forward through your shoulders until your legs lift off the floor. Keep your heels and big toes together, and your legs strong. Stay in the pose, breathing steadily. Exhale and lower your legs to the floor. Release your hands and relax in Devotional Pose (page 207).

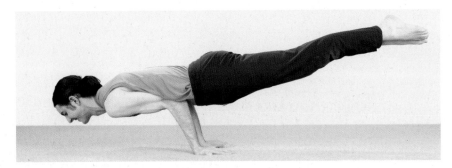

PEACOCK WITH LOTUS

1. Begin in Full Lotus (page 90). Inhale and roll forward into a modified Table Pose (page 23). Place your palms down with your fingertips toward your toes and your elbows in your solar plexus.

2. Strongly activate your abdominal muscles and lean forward through your shoulders until your legs lift off the floor. Keep your heels and big toes together, and your legs strong. Stay in the pose, breathing steadily.

3. Exhale and lower your legs to the floor. Release your hands and legs, and relax in Devotional Pose (page 207). Repeat by crossing your legs in Lotus with the opposite leg on top.

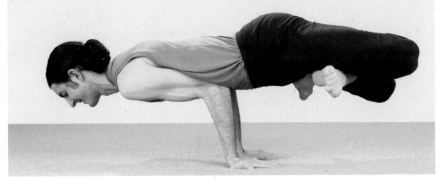

REVOLVED DOUBLE LEG FORWARD BEND

1. Begin sitting with both legs extended straight forward. Exhale, bend forward, and grasp your left big toe with your right hand.
2. Inhale, draw your left leg up to about 45 degrees. Position your spine as straight as possible.
3. Exhale, twist to the left and extend your left arm parallel to the floor. Rotate your head to gaze back at your left hand.
4. Inhale, release from the pose. Exhale, lower your arms and left leg. Repeat on the right side.

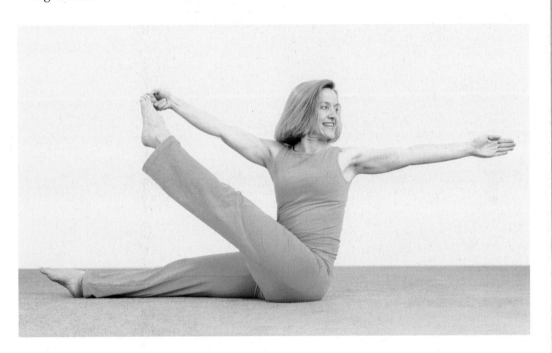

SIDE BOW

1. Begin resting on your right side. Position your right arm underneath your body. Tone your buttocks. Arch and reach back to grasp your right ankle.

2. Reach your left hand back for your left ankle. Adjust the position of your shoulders, spine, and hip in order to extend fully in the back bend. Draw your head back slightly as an extension of the stretch. Breathe steadily.

3. Exhale, release both legs and gently roll onto your stomach. Press back into Devotional Pose (page 207) to release tightness in your lower back. Repeat on the other side.

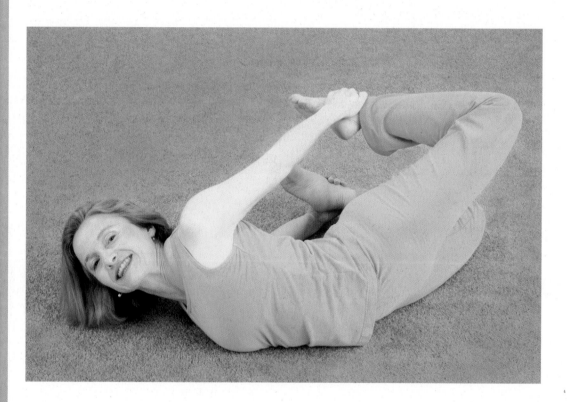

DRAWN BOW

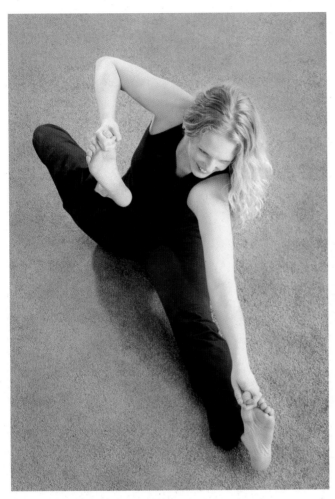

1. Begin sitting in Staff Pose (page 23) with both legs extended forward. Exhale, reach forward to catch your big toes using your first two fingers.

2. Inhale, activate your abdominal muscles, and bend your left leg. Draw your heel up to your left ear. Lift your left elbow as if drawing a bowstring. Your head remains centered and your gaze is toward your right big toe.

3. Hold the pose, breathing steadily. Exhale and release your left leg to the floor. Repeat on the other side.

Gaze:	Big toe on the extended leg.
Warm-ups:	Hip Cradle (page 22), Half Lotus (page 89), Half Spinal Twist (page 52), and Double Leg Forward Bend (page 42).
Counterposes:	Double Leg Forward Bend (page 42), Reclined Hip Rolls (page 54).
Easy variation:	Fold the extended leg in toward the body.
Benefits:	Creates a supple spine, open hip joints, flexible legs.

TORTOISE

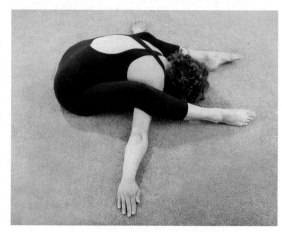

1. Begin sitting with your legs extended. Bend both legs by lifting the knees slightly. Position your feet about two feet apart. Exhale, bend forward and slide your arms underneath your knees.

2. Extend through the spine and bring your shoulders toward the floor. With your shoulders on the floor, your chin will rest comfortably on the floor as well.

3. Inhale, bend your legs, lift your shoulders, and draw your arms out from underneath your legs. Sit back up and extend your legs.

TORTOISE IN SHELL

1. Begin sitting with your legs extended. Bend both legs by lifting your knees slightly. Position your feet about two feet apart. Exhale, bend forward, and slide your arms underneath your knees.

2. Extend through your spine and bring your shoulders toward the floor. With your shoulders on the floor, tuck in your chin to rest your forehead on the floor as well.

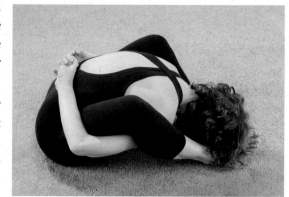

3. Cross your ankles right above your head or bring the soles of your feet together. Wrap your arms around your body to catch your hands behind your back. Relax your mind.

4. Exhale, release your arms and legs. Inhale, lift your shoulders.

Gaze:	Center of the forehead.
Warm-ups:	Sitting Straddle Forward Bend (page 46), Supine Cross-Legged Twist (page 205).
Counterposes:	Sitting Hip Rolls (page 199), twists.
Easy variation:	Single Leg Forward Bend (page 43), Shooting Star (page 200).
Breathing:	Inhale, lengthen your spine. Exhale into a Double Leg Forward Bend (page 42). Inhale, lift out of the pose. Exhale into the sitting posture.

REVERSE PLANK

1. Begin sitting in Staff Pose (page 23) with your legs extended and hands beside your hips. Inhale and activate your legs, buttocks, and abdomen.

2. Exhale, walk your hands under your shoulders with your fingers pointing to your toes, and lift. Bring your hips in line with your ankles, legs, and shoulders. Relax your head back behind your shoulders.

3. Exhale to release out of the posture by placing your hips on the floor.

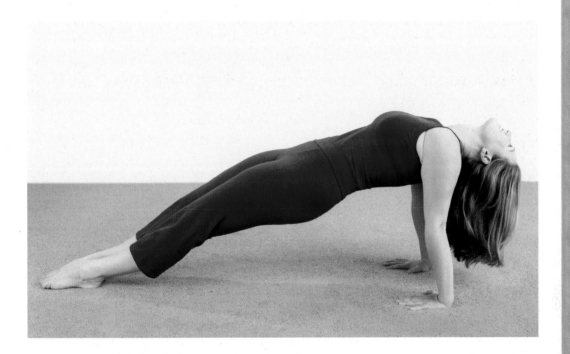

WHEEL, SOMERSAULT

1. Begin in Staff Pose (page 23) with your legs straight and hands on the sides of your hips. Exhale and extend your legs back over your head as in a somersault.

2. To roll through beyond your head and shoulders, press firmly down on your hands and straighten your arms. As your toes touch the floor, stabilize and come up into Downward Facing Dog (page 73).

3. To release, exhale into Devotional Pose (page 207).

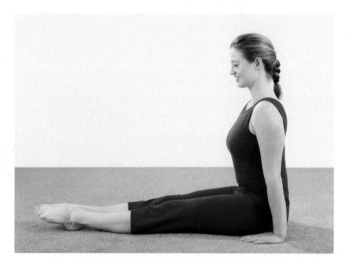

1

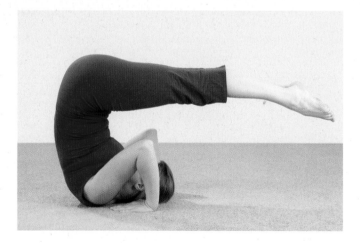

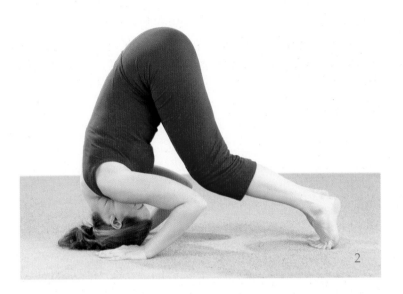

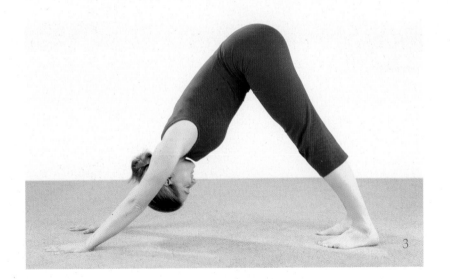

BRIDGE, STRAIGHT LEGS

1. Begin resting on the floor, face up. Activate your abdominal muscles. Bend both legs and place your feet parallel to each other underneath your knees.

2. Exhale, press your lower back to the floor. Tone your buttocks and inhale, lifting your hips. Draw your arms and shoulders underneath your body to support your hips. Place your hands under the boney crests of your hips. Extend fully in the back bend, breathing steadily.

3. Step your feet out slowly to straighten your legs. Bring your ankles together.

4. Exhale, releasing from the pose by stepping your feet underneath your knees. Release your hands and gently place each vertebra on the floor.

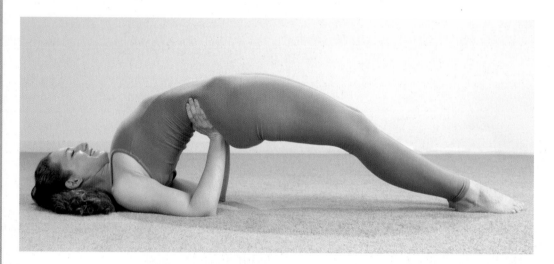

HEAD, ELBOWS ON FLOOR, STRAIGHT LEGS

1. Begin lying on the floor, face up. Bring your heels together and activate your legs. Tone your buttocks.

2. Place your hands on the floor in reverse next to your ears, fingertips underneath your shoulders and pointing toward your feet. Exhale and press your lower back to the floor. Inhale, lift your hips partway into a backbend with the crown of your head on the floor.

3. With the crown of your head remaining on the floor, place your right elbow underneath your shoulder. Then bring your left elbow to the floor underneath your shoulder. Straighten your legs. Arch, fully extending your spine and lifting your ribs.

4. To release, bend your legs, walking your feet underneath your knees as if practicing Bridge Pose (page 64). Exhale, tuck in your chin to rest the back of your head and shoulders on the floor. Rest your arms alongside your hips and stretch out flat.

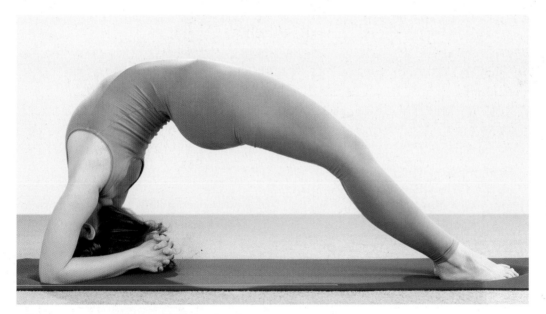

Gaze: Center of the forehead.
Warm-ups: Bridge Pose (page 64), Headstand (page 72), Upward Bow (page 128).
Counterposes: Wind Reliever (page 48), Reclined Hip Twist (page 22).
Easy variation: Bridge Pose (page 64).
Benefits: Strongly extends through the neck, shoulders, and spine.
Breathing: Exhale, press your lower back to the floor. Inhale, lift your hips and place your arms. Exhale, extend your legs. Release, inhale and bend your legs, stepping your feet in toward your body. Exhale, lower your spine.

ARM BALANCE WITH SCISSOR LEGS

1. Begin in a squat. Strongly rotate your legs to the left. Draw both knees up to rest on your left elbow.

2. Slowly scissor your legs. Extend your right leg (the lower leg) to the left. Extend your left leg (the top leg) straight out behind. Keep your breath steady. Repeat on the other side.

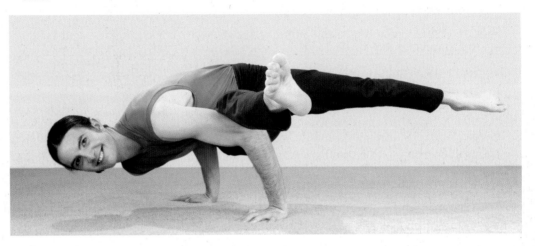

ARM BALANCE WITH SOLES OF FEET TOUCHING

1. Begin in a squat. Place your hands on the floor, shoulder distance apart. Wrap your legs around your elbows. Slide your knees as far up toward your shoulder joints as possible. Activate your abdominal muscles.

2. Transfer your weight onto your hands and lift into the balance position. Touch the soles of your feet together.

3. Exhale and release out of the pose. Massage your wrists and forearms to relax them.

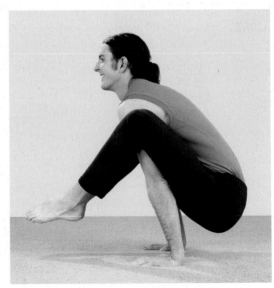

ARM BALANCE WITH ANKLES HOOKED

1. Begin in a squat. Place your hands on the floor, shoulder distance apart. Wrap your legs around your elbows. Slide your knees as far up toward your shoulder joints as possible. Activate your abdominal muscles.

2. Transfer your weight onto your hands, and lift into the balance position. Hook your ankles together.

3. Exhale to release out of the pose. Massage your wrists and forearms to relax them.

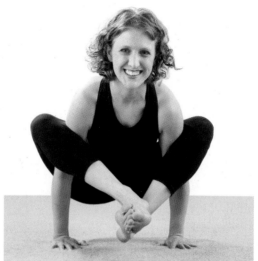

ARM BALANCE WITH ANKLES CROSSED AROUND ARM

1. Begin in Table Pose (page 23). Widen the distance between your hands. Draw your right leg over your right arm as high up as possible. Bring your left leg forward and hook your legs at the ankles. Tip to the left side, raising your legs to the right. Squeeze your legs in toward each other and keep your right hip lifted.

2. Exhale, release your legs, and rest in Devotional Pose (page 207).

3. Repeat on the other side.

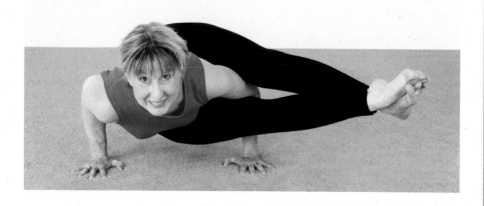

HEADSTAND WITH HANDS SUPPORTING

1. Begin in Devotional Pose (page 207). Position your head on the floor. Place your hands on the floor, palms down and shoulder distance apart, about a foot from your head. Inhale and kick your legs straight up. Activate your whole body. Keep your ankles and toes together.

2. Exhale and roll your legs down. Remain in Devotional Pose (page 207) a few moments.

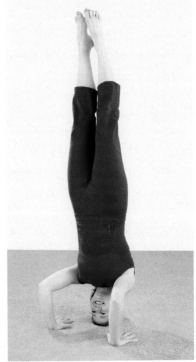

HEADSTAND WITH LEGS PARALLEL TO THE FLOOR (PIKE HEADSTAND)

1. Begin in Devotional Pose (page 207). Position your head on the floor. Place your hands on the floor, palms down and shoulder distance apart, about a foot from your head.

2. Inhale, straighten and tone your legs. Activate your abdominal muscles and slowly raise your legs so they are parallel to the floor. Keep your ankles and toes together.

3. Exhale and slowly lower your legs. Remain in Devotional Pose (page 207) a few moments.

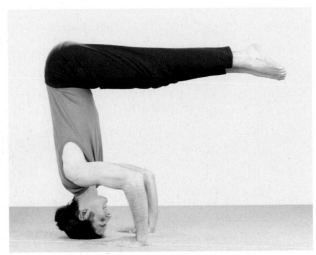

HEADSTAND WITH LOTUS

1. Begin in Headstand (page 72). To get into Full Lotus (page 90), fold your right leg and rest your foot on your left thigh. Then place your left foot on your right thigh. Tuck in your pelvis and press your knees up toward the ceiling in order to lengthen your spine.

2. Exhale, release from the pose. Stay in Devotional Pose (page 207) for a few moments. Repeat with your legs crossed in reverse.

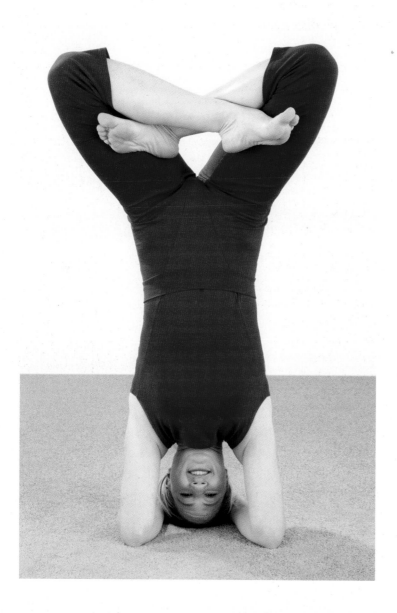

Home Practices

Full Yogic Breath

This three-part inhalation and three-part exhalation deeply purifies as it relaxes. The breath can be practiced either sitting or resting on your back. (It is easiest to learn resting on your back.)

Stretch out on the floor and begin with your hands resting on the sides of your hips. Breathe in, expanding your abdomen to a count of three, then expand your stomach, counting to three; complete the breath by expanding your upper chest, counting to three. Pause, retaining the breath, and count to three. Exhale completely first from your upper chest, counting to three, then from your stomach, counting to three, and finally from your abdomen, counting to three. Pause for a count of three before beginning the next breath cycle.

The pause between the breath cycles holds a special significance in yogic practice. It is the space where there is pure awareness. Therefore, bring your attention to this moment between the inhalation and the exhalation.

Find your own appropriate rhythm by adjusting the count more than or less than three. Don't hold the breath to the point where you feel tense. Just allow the breath energy to move fluidly through your body. Try this breathing exercise three times before relaxing into your regular breath.

Meditation on OM Namah Shivaya

OM Namah Shivaya means, "I bow down with respect to my Inner Self." It is an ancient mantra that has been repeated by many sages throughout time. The mantra OM Namah Shivaya is a living force. Its power emanates directly from the Inner Self and, when you repeat it with consciousness and devotion, it is possible to experience the Self. On the most basic level, when you sit and begin to meditate, you should just be repeating "OM Namah Shivaya" with the inhalation and the exhalation, not hard or fast, just in a natural way. Tie the mantra to the breath. As you repeat the mantra, your mind is going to start thinking. That's okay. Don't start judging yourself. Just let go of the thoughts and bring awareness back to OM Namah Shivaya.

Hatha Yoga Practice Sequence

Sun Salutation, Easy (Surya namaskar), pages 76-77,
  with Cobra (Bhujangasana), page XX

Sun Salutation, Aerobic (Surya namaskar), pages 78-79, with Upward Facing Dog
  (Urdhva Mukha Svanasana), page 67

Shambhava leg and hip stretches, pages 202-205

Upward Facing Double Leg Forward Bend I (Urdhva Mukha Paschimottanasana I),
  page 151

Upward Facing Double Leg Forward Bend II (Urdhva Mukha Paschimottanasana II),
  page 152

Heron (Krounchasana), page 153

Heron (Krounchasana) with Half Lotus (Ardha Padmasana), page 153

Twist with Hands Behind the Back (Marichyasana), page 104

Arm Balance with Ankles Hooked (Bhujapidasana), page 171

Drawn Bow (Akarna Dhanurasana), page 163

Tortoise (Kurmasana), page 164

Double Leg Wind Reliever (Apanasana), page 205

Reclined Hip Rolls, page 22

Savasana, page 206

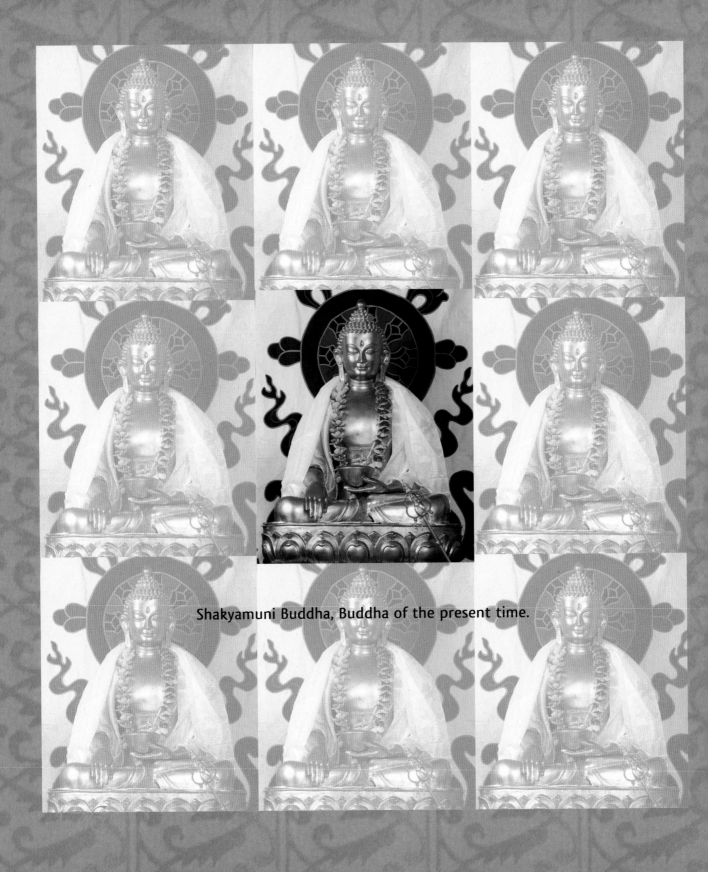

Shakyamuni Buddha, Buddha of the present time.

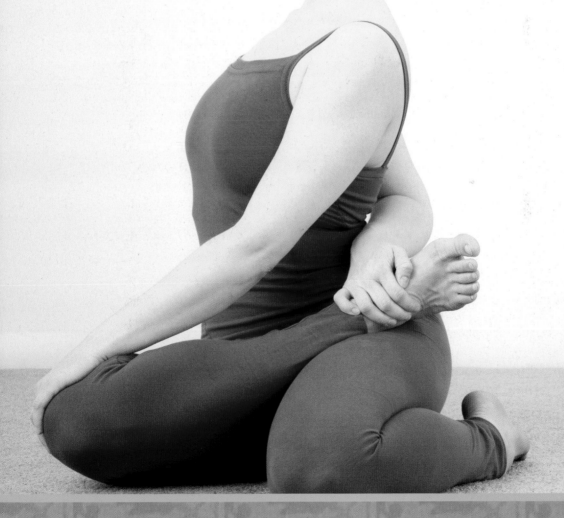

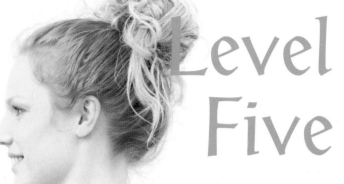
Level Five

Postures

Chapter Five

Level Five Postures

"The heart is the hub of all holy places. Go there and roam."
– Bhagavan Nityananda

STANDING GARLAND POSE

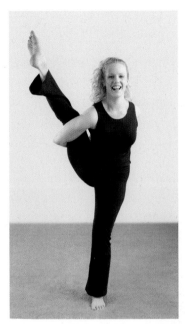

1. Begin in Mountain (page 26). Shift onto your left foot and draw your right leg up, knee to chest. Keep your knee high and shift it behind your shoulder. Catch your hands under your right thigh with your left hand wrapping behind your hip.

2. As this is a strong balance pose, make sure your breath is deep and full. Release from the pose. Exhale and release your foot to the floor, relaxing your arms. Switch sides and repeat the pose.

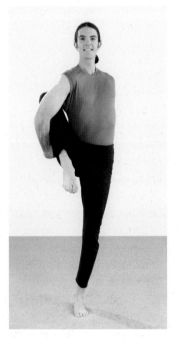

VARIATION 1

1. For variation, keep your right knee high and wrap your arms around your knee. Your right arm will reach forward and around. Your left arm will reach behind your ribs to catch your right hand.

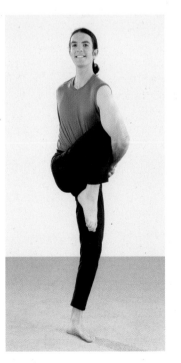

VARIATION 2

1. For another variation, keep your right knee high and draw it over to your left shoulder. Wrap your left arm around your knee and right arm behind your back to catch your hands.

NOOSE

1. Begin in a squat position with both feet flat.
2. Exhale, rotate left. Swing your arms around your knees to catch your hands behind your back.
3. Inhale, lengthen your spine. Exhale, look over your left shoulder.
4. Inhale, release from the twist. Exhale, release your hands. Repeat on the other side.

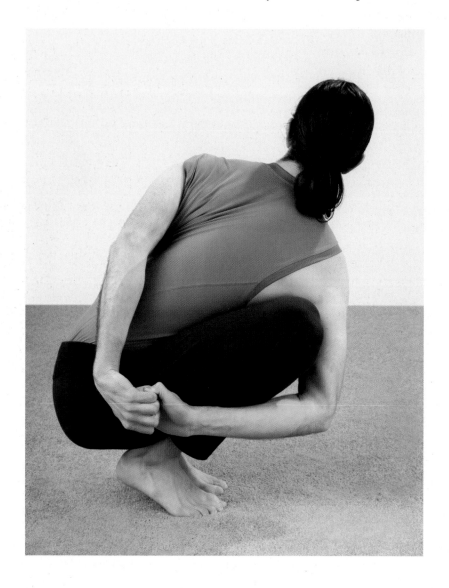

DANCER, FULL POSE

1. Begin standing in Mountain (page 26). Shift your weight onto your left leg and raise your right heel to your buttock. Reach back and grasp your right big toe with your right hand. Inhale and arch your back, lifting your leg up higher and drawing your elbow out to the side and up over your shoulder. Move carefully without forcing any movement.

2. Reach your left arm up over your shoulder and grasp your right big toe. Keep extending through your heart, chest, and spine.

3. Exhale to gently release from the pose, repositioning your right foot on the floor.

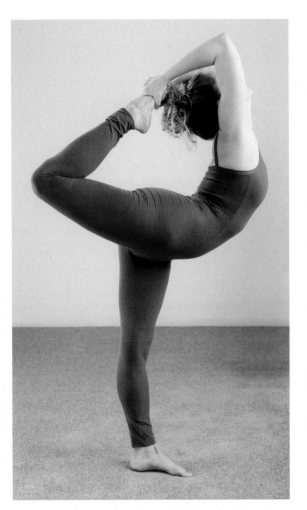

Gaze:	Center of the forehead.
Warm-ups:	Sitting Cradle Stretch (page 200), Camel (page 62), Upward Bow (page 128), Scissor Split (page 134).
Counterpose:	Catcher's Stretch (page 197).
Easy variation:	Do this reaching one hand back for your ankle.
Benefits:	Tones the back and shoulders; promotes hip flexibility; releases toxins.
Breathing:	Inhale, raise your leg, and bring one elbow over your shoulder. With the next inhalation, lift through your heart. Exhale, reach your second hand back for your toe. To release from the pose, exhale and gently lower your leg.

SITTING, ANKLE BEHIND HEAD

1. Begin sitting in Staff Pose (page 23) with both legs extended forward. Tone the abdominal muscles and reach for the lower left leg to cradle it. Draw the ankle up past the shoulder to rest behind the neck. Draw the left arm in front of the left leg. Bring the palms together in namaste. Lift the head so the chin is parallel to the floor. Keep the right leg strong and active.

2. Exhale to release the top leg. Switch sides.

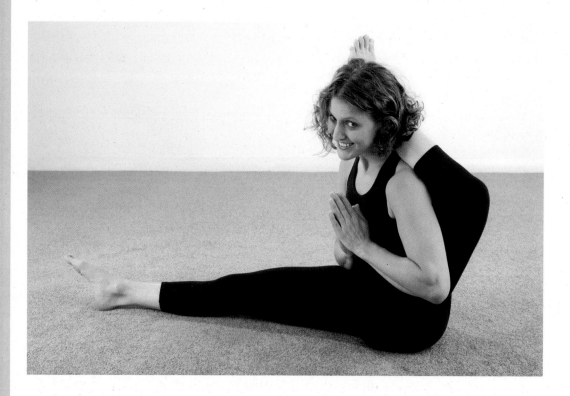

Gaze: Center of the forehead.

Warm-ups: Scissor Splits (page 134), Lunges (page 22), Pigeon Pose with One Leg Extended (page 68).

Counterposes: Wind Reliever (page 48), Reclined Hip Twist (page 22).

Easy variation: Sitting Cradle Stretch (page 200).

Benefits: Deep hip and leg stretch.

Breathing: From the floor, inhale and lift your leg. Exhale, release it behind your shoulder. Inhale and lift your shoulders. Exhale, release from the pose. Switch sides.

SITTING, ANKLE BEHIND HEAD FORWARD BEND

1. Practice Sitting, Ankle Behind Head (page 182). While in the upright sitting position, exhale into Forward Bend (page 43). Keep your ankle behind your neck and reach forward, extending your arms down the outstretched leg.

2. To release from the pose, inhale and raise your shoulders. Exhale and release your leg from your back. Stretch your feet out in Staff Pose (page 23).

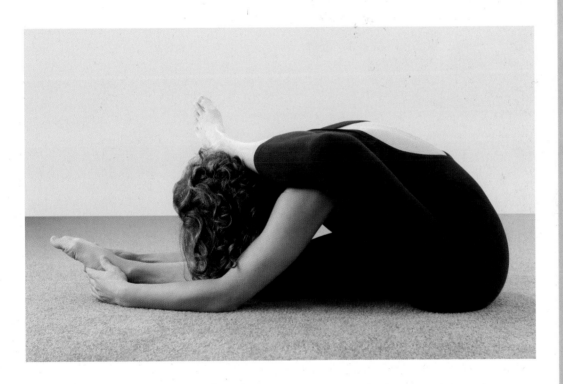

RECLINING, ANKLE BEHIND HEAD

1. Begin on your back with both feet on the floor. Cradle your left leg and place your left ankle behind your shoulder and neck. Stretch your right leg out across the floor. Bring your hands together in prayer pose. If your left leg is slipping, continue to hold it in place with your right hand.

2. Release from the pose by placing your right foot on the floor, then releasing your left leg. Relax your back, curling into Double Leg Wind Reliever (page 48). Repeat on the other side.

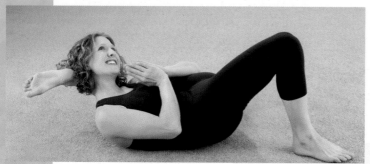

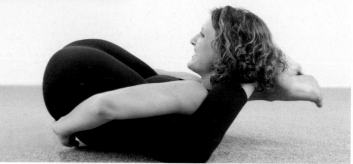

RECLINING, BOTH ANKLES BEHIND HEAD

1. Take your left leg and place your left ankle behind your neck. Stabilize your left leg by bringing your left arm in front of your leg. Place your right ankle behind your left ankle. Stabilize that leg by bringing your right arm in front of your leg. Your chin may rest comfortably on your collar bone. Bring your hands behind the back and clasp fingers underneath the hips. Breathe in a relaxed, even manner.

2. To release from the pose, uncross your ankles one at a time. Stretch out in Savasana (page 206). Practice Sitting Hip Rolls (page 199).

CRANE WITH LEG EXTENDED

1. From Crow Hand Balance (page 113), shift your weight to the right and inhale to extend your left leg. Keep your left leg in line with your torso and keep your body toned.

2. Exhale to release your left leg down. Drop your toes to the floor and assume a squat position.

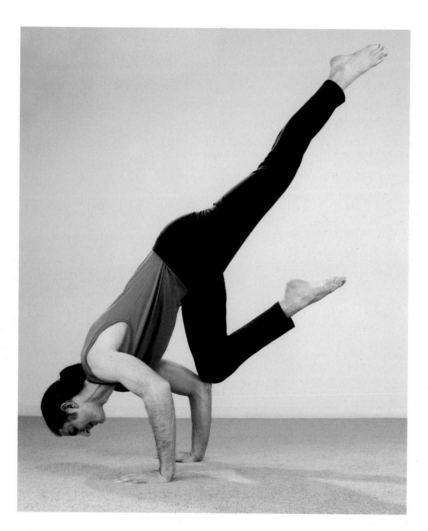

STRADDLE ARM BALANCE

1. Begin in a squat position. Place your hands on the floor, shoulder distance apart. Lift your knees up over your shoulders.

2. Transfer your weight onto your hands, and extend your legs forward and up in a straddle. Keep your legs as straight as possible.

3. If possible, lift your toes up above your shoulders.

4. Exhale, bend your legs, and relax back down to a sitting posture.

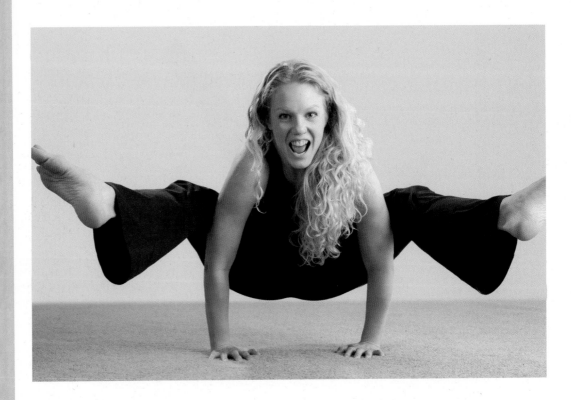

SCISSOR LEG ARM BALANCE II

1. Begin in a squat. Lunge your left knee forward and rest it on your left knee. Strongly engage your abdominal muscles.

2. Tip forward, transferring your weight onto your left knee. Scissoring the legs, extend your upper leg (the left leg) to the left. Extend you lower leg (the right leg) straight out behind. Keep the breath steady.

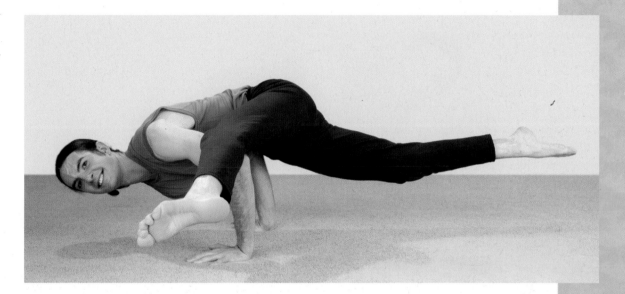

BOTH LEGS EXTENDED TO SIDE

1. Begin in a squat. Strongly rotate the legs to the left. Draw both knees up to rest on the left elbow.

2. Tip forward. Slowly extend both of the legs to the left. Keep the breath steady.

3. Repeat on the other side.

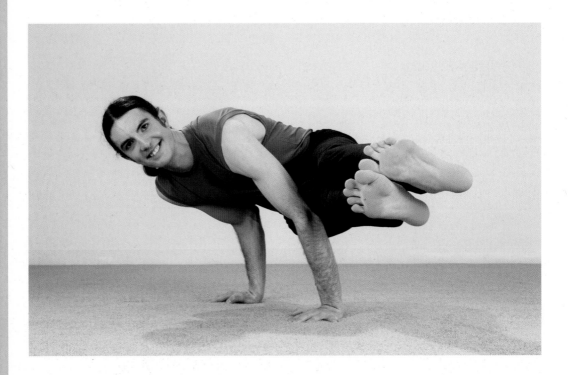

SPLIT SIDE PLANK

1. Begin in a lunge with your left leg forward. Exhale and lean into the lunge to place your left hand on the floor inside your left leg.

2. Press down through your left hand and activate your abdominal muscles. Lean your left leg on your left shoulder and raise your lower left leg as if in a split. Keep pressing your left leg into your arm and shoulder to maintain the posture.

3. Exhale to release from the pose. Repeat on the other side

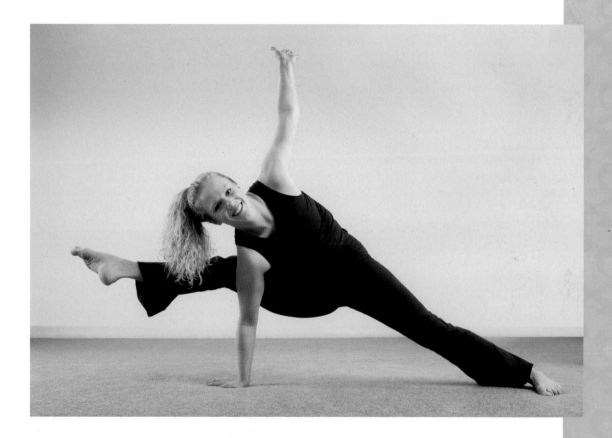

SIDE PLANK
ANKLE BEHIND HEAD

1. Begin in Sitting, Ankle Behind Head Forward Bend (page 183), sitting with your left ankle behind your neck. Lean to the left side, and carefully move into a side lunge with your left leg still supported on your shoulder and your ankle behind your neck.

2. Exhale and lean into the lunge. Press down through your left hand and activate your abdominal muscles.

3. Lift your head and chest. Raise your top arm straight upward.

4. Keep pressing your left leg into your shoulder to maintain the posture.

5. Exhale to release from the pose, carefully tucking your chin in and lowering your hips to the floor. Release your leg.

6. Repeat on the other side.

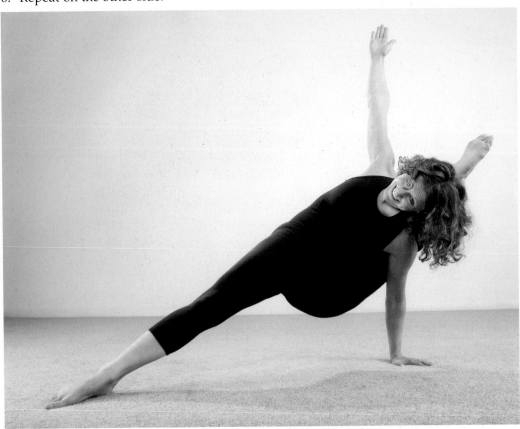

FOREARM BALANCE
WITH FULL CURL

1. Begin in Devotional Pose (page 207). Stretch your arms out across the floor, shoulder distance apart. Keep your elbows shoulder distance apart. Activate your arms and shoulders.

2. Pressing on your forearms, exhale to kick up into Forearm Balance (page 143). Begin with a gentle curve throughout your spine. Tone your torso, buttocks, and legs. Keep your heels toward each other. Position your head so that your face is toward the floor. Gently gaze at the point between your eyebrows. Your shoulder joints will be over your elbows.

3. When your balance is steady, continue to extend your spine further. Bring your toes to touch the crown of your head.

4. Exhale, release from the pose, and lower your feet to the floor. Stay in Devotional Pose (page 207) for a few breaths.

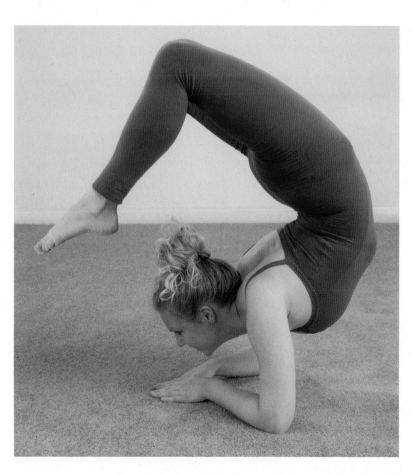

Home Practices

Robin's Breath

This is a gentle, heart-opening, and energizing breathing sequence. Begin sitting comfortably with palms together at the heart. Breathe in deeply, enjoying the breath. Exhale, extend both arms straight forward with the palms together. Inhale, separate the palms out to the T-position and continue the stretch, arching and drawing the arms back as far as possible. Exhale, relax the arms, bringing the palms straight forward and together again, tuck the chin, and round the upper back. Inhale, bring the palms back to the heart.

Sipping Breath

This breathing exercise energizes you just as a brisk walk would. Begin sitting comfortably with palms together at the heart. Breathe in deeply through the nose allowing the abdomen to expand. Exhale through the nose, and round the spine, dropping the head toward the floor. Raise the body back up in six steps, taking a light sipping breath through the nostrils each time. Repeat this three times and then sit quietly to absorb the energy.

Gratitude Meditation

Begin sitting comfortably with palms together at the heart. Cup the hands together at the center of the chest, the heart chakra, with the fingers pointing upward. Breathing through the nose, take a breath into the heart center. Hold the breath in the heart, and feel sweetness and love well up. Keeping the base of the palms together, let the fingertips come apart like a lotus flower opening as it blooms.

See this as an expansiveness of love and an expression of the overflowing love in your heart. Raise this flower and your hands heavenward. As the hands rise higher, the palms separate and the arms reach upward and outward to the sides above your head. The shape of your arms becomes like a huge bowl with the base at the heart. Feel your love, gratitude, and all the sweetness in your heart being offered upward.

Make a gift of love and thanks to your teachers, Gurus, and the enlightened beings of all times for the tremendous opportunity to be alive and to be able to grow and to do spiritual practice. Feel gratitude for their help and assistance. Feel a sense of humility. Offer all these upward. With the exhale, you can let your hands rest back down into your lap.

Hatha Yoga Practice Sequence

Sun Salutation, Easy (Surya Namaskar), pages 76-77, with Cobra (Bhujangasana), page 56

Sun Salutation, Aerobic (Surya Namaskar), pages 78-79, with Upward Facing Dog (Urdhva Mukha Svanasana), page 67

Shambhava yoga leg and hip stretches, pages 202-205

Standing Garland Pose and variation (Eka Pada Malasana), page 179

Noose (Pasasana), page 180

Half Lotus (Ardha Padmasana), page 89

Sitting, Ankle Behind Head (Skandasana), page 182

Sitting, Ankle Behind Head Forward Bend (Skandasana with Forward Bend), page 183

Straddle Arm Balance (Tittibhasana), page 186

Split Side Plank (Vishvamitrasana), page 189

Forearm Balance with Full Curl (Vrschikasana), page 191

Devotional Pose (Bhaktasana), page 207

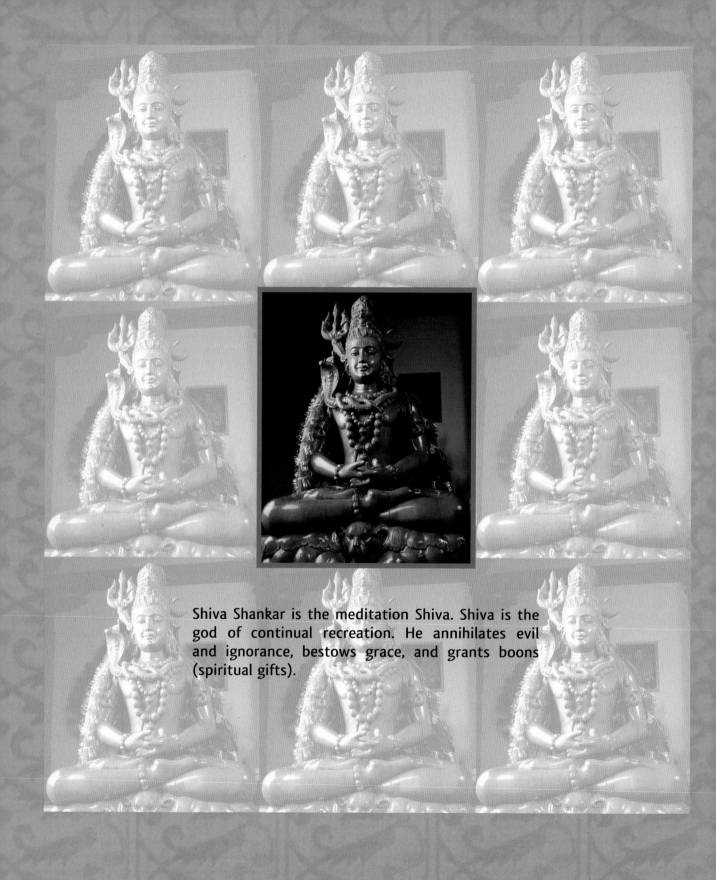

Shiva Shankar is the meditation Shiva. Shiva is the god of continual recreation. He annihilates evil and ignorance, bestows grace, and grants boons (spiritual gifts).

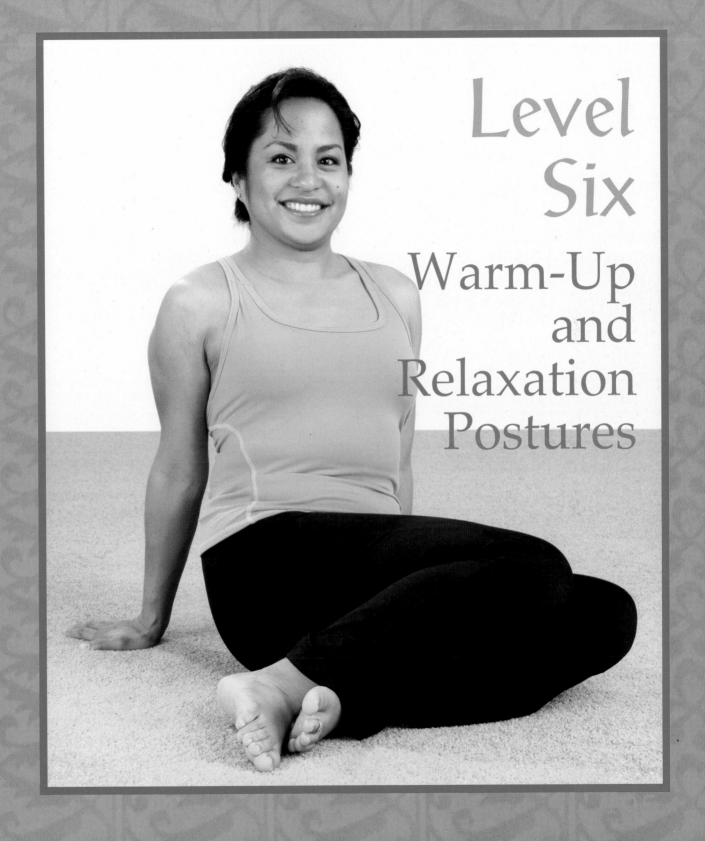

Level
Six

Warm-Up
and
Relaxation
Postures

Chapter Six

Warm-Up and Relaxation Postures

*"Inside of you is a state of being that is
totally pure and clear and at peace."*
—*Sri. Shambhavananda*

TWISTING BEAR

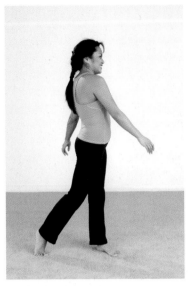

1. Begin in Mountain (page 26) and let your arms swing gently from side to side. Lift your back heel when turning to the opposite side.

SHOULDER STRETCH AGAINST WALL

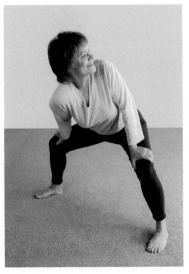

1. Begin standing with one of your shoulders to the wall. Place your feet one foot's length apart.

2. Stretch your inside arm up parallel to the floor. Place your outside hand against the wall at shoulder level.

3. Gently press into the stretch to open up your whole shoulder area. Release and repeat on the other side.

CATCHER'S STRETCH

1. Begin in Mountain (page 26) and position your feet three feet apart. Place your hands on your knees.

2. Exhale, drop your left shoulder forward while twisting right. Look over your right shoulder and breathe deeply, relaxing your belly.

3. Inhale back to center. Exhale, twist to the other side.

QUAD STRETCH AT WALL

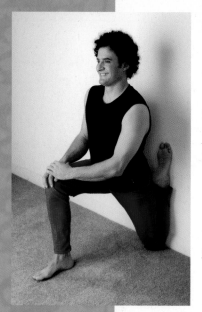

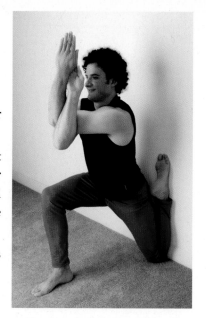

1. Begin in Table Pose (page 23) with your toes against the wall.
2. Lean right, inhale, and step your left foot forward, with your ankle below your knee. Slide your right foot up the wall and your right knee back against the baseboard.
3. On the next inhalation, lift your shoulders and place your hands on your knees.

4. Inhale and stretch your arms to a T-position. Exhale and criss-cross your right arm over your left at the elbow. Intertwine your forearms. Bring your palms together.
5. Exhale, lower your shoulders, and release from the stretch. Repeat on the other side.

CAT

COW

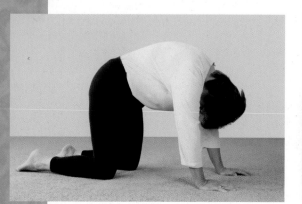

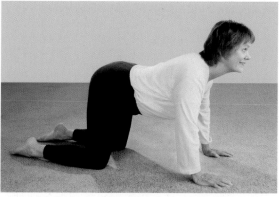

1. Begin in Table Pose (page 23). Arch your back with your shoulders toward the ceiling. Draw your abdominal muscles toward your spine.

1. Begin in Table Pose (page 23). Arch your back and lower your abdomen toward the floor. Lift your head toward the ceiling.

RABBIT

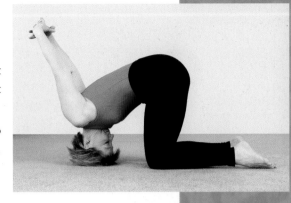

1. Begin in Devotional Pose (page 207). Clasp your hands at the base of your spine. Place your forehead right in front of your knees. Curl your toes underneath your heels.

2. Inhale, lift your hips and roll forward, massaging the top of your head. Draw your arms high over your shoulders.

3. Exhale, release back to Devotional Pose (page 207).

BUTTERFLY

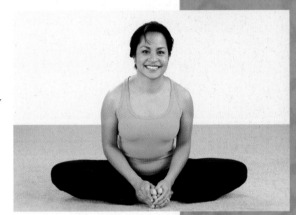

1. Begin sitting with the soles of your feet together. Draw your heels close to the base of your body.

2. Breathing steadily, lift and lower your legs.

SITTING HIP ROLLS

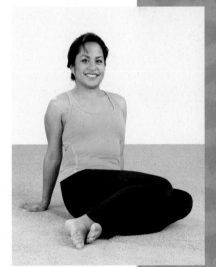

1. Begin sitting with your knees drawn up to your body and your feet on the floor.

2. Moving easily with the breath, roll both knees from side to side.

SITTING CRADLE STRETCH

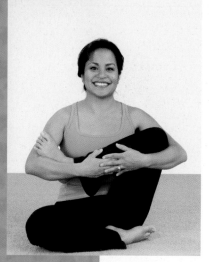

1. Begin sitting with your legs crossed. Lift your right foot up to cradle it between your elbows.

2. Move with the breath. Exhale to lower your leg. Repeat on the other side.

SHOOTING STAR, RELAXING FORWARD BEND

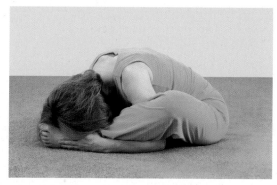

1. Begin with your legs crossed. Bring the soles of your feet together, placed a body length away from the base of your body.

2. Let your knees drop out to your sides. Exhale, round forward, and scoop both arms underneath your legs. Rest your hands on top of your feet.

3. Inhale, raise your shoulders to come out of the pose.

PLANK

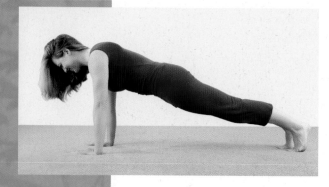

1. Begin in Table Pose (page 23). Lean onto your hands and lock your elbows. Tone your abdomen and step your legs out behind to straighten them. Tone your legs and keep your ankles side by side. Align your head, neck, spine, and legs.

2. Exhale out of the pose and rest in Devotional Pose (page 207).

CHATURANGA

1. Begin lying face down on the mat. Place your hands underneath your shoulders and curl your toes under. Inhale and lift your body up a few inches off the floor. Keep your shoulders, hips, and heels aligned. Remain in the pose with the breath steady.

2. Exhale, release from the pose, and rest on the mat. Turn your head to one side.

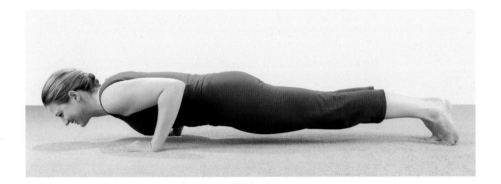

EASY UPWARD FACING DOG

1. Begin in Devotional Pose (page 207) with your arms stretched forward across the floor. Inhale, launch forward and up, resting on your hands and locking your elbows. Gently extend through your spine, keeping your knees on the floor. Lift your feet to bring your toes toward each other. Lift through your upper chest.

2. Exhale, release out of the pose. Rest in Devotional Pose (page 207).

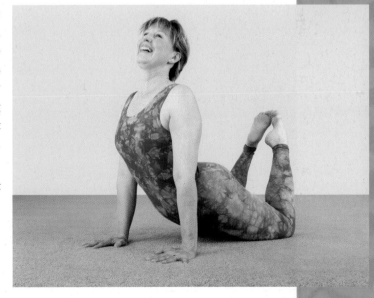

WIND RELIEVER

1. Begin lying on your back, stretched out across the floor. Bend your right leg to catch your hands around your right knee. Inhale, draw your knee toward your shoulder.

2. Exhale and curl up, bringing your cheek toward your knee.

3. Inhale, relax your back to the floor.

4. Exhale, release your knee. Repeat on the left side.

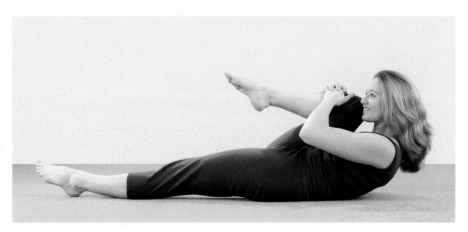

FIGURE 4

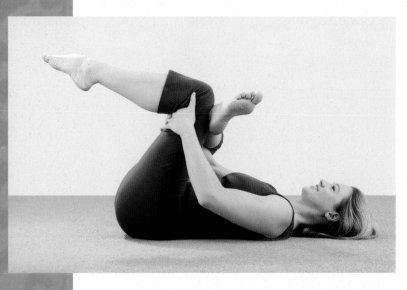

1. Begin lying on your back. Bend your left leg, placing your foot on the floor underneath your knee. Rest your right ankle on your left knee.

2. Curl forward, sliding your right arm underneath your right leg in order to catch your hands around your left knee.

3. Rest your head and shoulders on the floor, and gently draw your left knee in toward your shoulder.

4. Exhale, release the stretch, and repeat on the other side.

SUPINE CRADLE

1. Begin resting on the floor with your spine extended. Exhale, curl forward to cradle your lower right leg in your arms between your elbows.

2. Extend your left leg straight out and gaze at your left toes. Your left leg will be six inches above the floor. Keep the breath steady.

3. Exhale, release from the pose. Repeat on the other side.

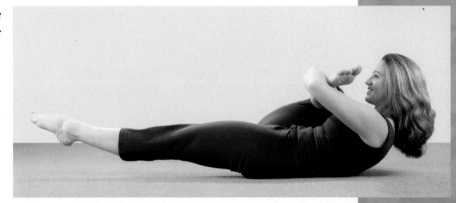

SUPINE LEG EXTENSION VERTICAL

1. Begin resting on the floor. Bend your right leg and hold your leg behind your calf. Inhale, stretch your leg straight up above your hip.

2. Exhale to release and repeat on the other side.

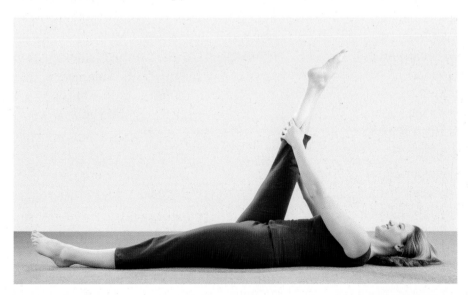

SUPINE LEG EXTENSION CROSS TO OPPOSITE SIDE

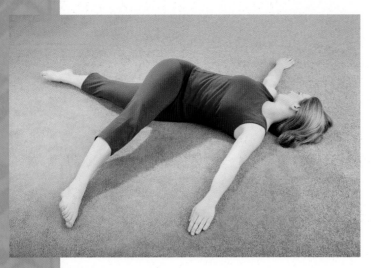

1. Begin resting on the floor with your arms in the T-position. Inhale, stretch your right leg straight up above your hip. Exhale, rotate your leg to the left. If possible, bring your right foot to the floor. Rotate your head to the right.

2. Inhale, raise your leg back up above your hip. Exhale, release your leg to the floor. Repeat on the other side.

SUPINE LEG EXTENSION TO OPEN SIDE

1. Begin resting on the floor with your arms in the T-position. Inhale, stretch your right leg straight up above your hip. Exhale, rotate your leg to the right. If possible, bring your right foot to the floor. Rotate your head to the left.

2. Inhale, raise your right leg back up above your hip. Exhale, release your leg to the floor. Repeat on the other side.

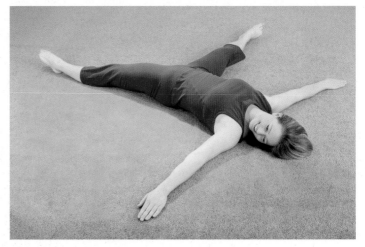

SUPINE CROSS-LEGGED TWIST

1. Begin resting on the floor with your knees bent and both feet underneath your knees. Position your arms on the floor in the T-position.

2. Cross your right leg over your left leg. Exhale, roll your knees down to the left. Rotate your head right and gaze at your right hand.

3. Inhale, lift your knees back to center. Exhale, release your legs, and repeat on the other side.

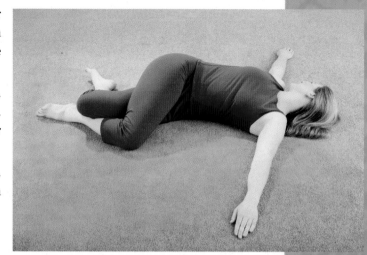

DOUBLE LEG WIND RELIEVER

1. Begin resting on the floor. Catch your hands around both knees. Exhale, bring your forehead toward your knees.

2. Inhale, relax your head to the floor. Exhale, relax your knees over your hips. Repeat three times.

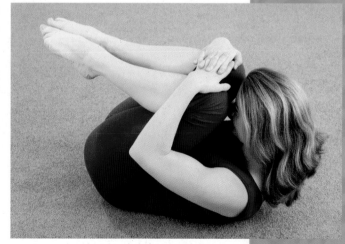

SAVASANA

1. Begin resting on the floor, face up. Position your ankles about hip distance apart. Let your feet relax and your toes fall out to the sides. Position your arms about six inches from the side of your hips. Relax your hands with palms up.

2. Relax your face and eyes. Breathe deeply to relax completely.

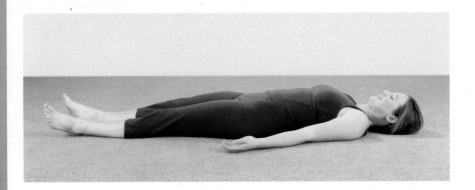

DOWNWARD FACING SAVASANA

1. Rest face down, stretched out on the floor. Position your hands palms up, six inches from the side of your hips. Position your feet a comfortable distance apart. Turn your head to one side. Breathe in a relaxed manner.

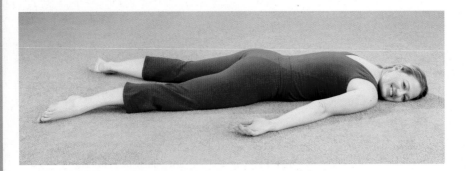

DEVOTIONAL POSE (BHAKTASANA)

1. Begin kneeling with your ankles hip distance apart and lower your hips to rest on your heels. Stretch your arms forward, palms down. Breathe deeply to relax your hips, back, and shoulders.

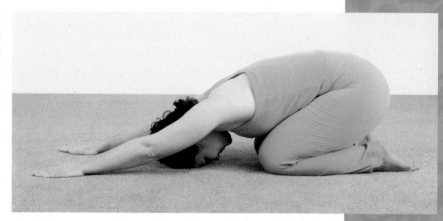

CHILD'S POSE

1. Begin kneeling with your ankles hip distance apart and lower your hips to rest on your heels. Stretch your arms back so your hands can cover your feet, palms down. Breathe deeply to relax your hips, back, and shoulders.

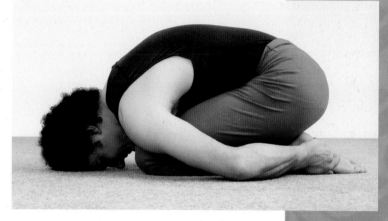

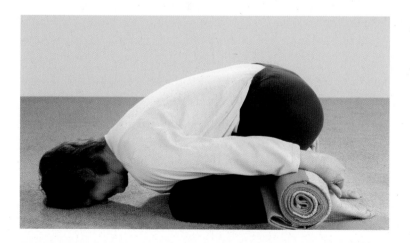

Supported Child's Pose

Home Practice Sequences

Gentle Face and Sinus Massage

1. With your thumbs, massage the inside edges of your eyebrows.

2. With your third fingers, massage the center of your eyebrow ridges, right over the brow hairs.

3. With your pinky fingers, massage the outside of the eyebrows.

4. With your thumbs side by side, massage your forehead right above your eyebrows. Slide up one inch and massage your forehead. Again, slide up one more inch and massage your forehead.

5. Massage your temples.

6. With your elbows lifted to the sides, massage your cheek crease, placing the first three fingers in the crease from the corners of your nose to the corners of your mouth.

7. With your index fingers, massage the center of your chin.

8. With your index fingers, massage your lower lip, then your upper lip, placing your fingers one third of the way along your lip line.

9. With your index fingers, massage the corners of your nose.

10. With your index fingers, massage halfway along the bridge of your nose, where the cartilage begins.

11. With your thumbs, press into the pressure points at the inside corners of your eye sockets, along the bridge of your nose.

12. Rub both hands together and place your warm hands over your eyes.

13. End with a nice deep breath.

Relaxation Visualization

1. Begin resting comfortably on the floor. Use a rolled yoga mat underneath your knees, a pillow behind your head or a rolled towel underneath your neck, and a blanket on top for warmth.

2. Relax, smile gently, and breathe deeply to release the surface tensions of the day. Visualize pleasant surroundings, and feel content and at peace.

3. Begin at your feet, visualizing a globe of white light underneath the arch of each foot. Gently absorb the white light and see it ascending to encompass your ankles. The light is soft and yet radiant. It absorbs heaviness, dullness, or discomfort.

4. Visualize the light lifting to your knees, and massaging your joints and tendons.

5. Visualize the light streams joining at your hips and lower spine. See the light brighten as the two streams join.

6. From your lower spine, visualize the light moving step by step up your spine, massaging the vertebrae, muscles, and nerves. See a delicate lotus light flower with the petals turned upward between each segment of your spine.

7. Allow the light to massage your neck and shoulders, and flow down both arms to your fingertips and hands.

8. Visualize the light lifting higher up to the top of your head. Visualize it cascading down across your forehead, chest, torso, and legs, back to your feet.

9. See yourself surrounded in the brilliant healing light. Absorb the light into every cell. Energize the visualization with the breath. Release heaviness with the exhalations.

10. Feel contentment and peace.

11. Take three deep breaths to begin to come out of the relaxation. Stretch your arms over your shoulders and from your toes to your shoulders. Take one more deep breath and yawn.

12. Roll onto one side. Supported by your hands, lift back up to a sitting position.

13. Take the relaxation and peacefulness with you.

Relax and Rejuvenate

A (20 minutes)

Prop legs and feet against the wall (3 minutes)

Shambhava leg and hip stretches (pages 202-205) (10 minutes)

Butterfly, page 199 (1 minute)

Sitting Cradle Stretch, page 200 (1 minute)

Savasana, page 206, to relax (5 minutes)

B (19 minutes)

Twisting Bear, page 197 (1 minute)

Staff of Brahma, page 74, (2 minutes)

Catcher's Stretch, page 197 (1 minute)

Quad Stretch at Wall, page 198 (1 minute)

Shambhava leg and hip stretches (pages 202-205) (10 minutes)

Savasana, page 206 (5 minutes)

Glossary

ACHARYA: Respected teacher

AJNA: The center of the forehead or the spiritual center between the eyebrows

ANAHATA: The heart center or the spiritual center in the center of the chest

ASANA: Seat or cushion for meditation. Also, postures practiced to strengthen muscles and nerves.

ASHRAM: Spiritual center, usually specific to a particular lineage of teachers; abode of a saint where spiritual disciplines are practiced

AYURVEDA: Knowledge of health; yogic path of self-healing

BABAJI: Term of endearment for a holy man ("baba" means father)

BHAGAWAN: One who is divine

BRAHMA: The first of the Hindu trinity and god of creation

CHAKRA: Spiritual energy center

DEITY: A god or goddess representing an aspect of divine consciousness

DEVOTION: Love for god

DHARANA: Focusing the mind and will

DHARMA: Essential duty; religious teachings

DHYANA: Concentrating awareness on the highest energies

DIKSHA: Blessings and spiritual initiation

DIVINE: God-like in nature

DRISTI: Gaze. In hatha yoga, the gaze directs the energy of vision in a posture.

DURGA: Goddess who rides on a lion or tiger; one who dispels all confusion

EGO: The limited "I" consciousness preoccupied with things such as the body, mind, and personality

FIRE CEREMONY: Sacred purification ceremony using mantras, yantras, fire, and masala offerings to establish harmony, happiness, and well-being for individuals, regions, and the world

GANESHA: Elephant-headed deity; Remover of obstacles and lord of compassion

GANESHPURI: Town in Maharastra where Bhagavan Nityananda and Baba Muktananda established spiritual centers; ancient place of worship

GURU: One who bestows the highest blessings; one who, having attained the highest realization, initiates others and guides them on the path to realization

Ham sah: Natural mantra of the Self that corresponds to the repetition of the breath: "I am divine consciousness"

Hatha yoga: Physical discipline of postures to purify the nervous system

Ida: The left nadi corresponding to the spinal region that is associated with feminine and cooling energy

Japa: Silent mantra repetition

Jiva: Individual soul

Karma: Actions, thoughts, and spoken words as related to the law of cause and effect

Kashmir Saivism: Branch of Hinduism with an emphasis on worshipping Shiva and on imparting knowledge via the heart connection between students and teacher. The teachings of Kashmir Saivism are revelations from Shiva known as the Shiva Sutras.

Krishna: Light-hearted aspect of the divine; flute player and eighth incarnation of Vishnu

Kundalini: Spiritual energy that, once awakened, purifies one's entire being

Lakshmi: Goddess of wealth and abundance on both spiritual and material planes; consort of Vishnu

Lineage: The continuum of masters who hold and also pass on the teachings of a spiritual tradition

Lingam: Unmanifest form of Shiva represented by a pillar of stone

Mahasamadhi: Literally, the great liberation. The liberation of saints from their bodies.

Mala: 108 beads strung together; used to focus the mind and to count mantra repetitions

Manipura: The third chakra; spiritual energy center located at the navel center

Mantra: Divine sounds imbued with transforming and protecting powers

Muladhara: The first chakra; spiritual energy center located at the base of the spine

Muktananda: Great meditation master and devotee of Bhagavan Nityananda. Muktananda established an ashram in Ganeshpuri, India; taught all over the world; and designed a weekend meditation intensive program for Westerners to receive deep spiritual transmissions.

Mukti: Liberation

Nadi: Subtle body channel that conducts spiritual energy

Nataraja: Creative, dancing aspect of Shiva surrounded by a ring of flames

Nityananda: Great saint, enlightened from a young age, who was the Guru of Muktananda and Rudrananda

OM: Primordial sound; the sound of the Self; sound from which everything manifests

OM Namah Shivaya: Great mantra "I bow to Shiva" or "I bow to the inner Self"

OM Gam Ganeshaya Namaha: Mantra of Lord Ganesha that helps to alleviate obstacles

Pancha Ganapati: The five-headed form of Ganesha

Patanjali: Credited with the Yoga Sutras, teachings and works on Ayurveda

Pingala: The right nadi corresponding to the spinal region; associated with masculine heating energy

Prana: Vital life force

Pranayama: Discipline of regulating the breath in order to produce certain results

Puja: Chanting worship in Sanskrit performed before a deity or saint

Rishi: Seer, one whose inner eye is fully opened through the process of meditation

Rudrananda: Great master of Kundalini meditation, Shambhavananda's first Guru

Sadhana: Spiritual practices undertaken on the spiritual path

Samadhi: State of enlightenment

Samsara: Cycles of death and rebirth

Sangha: Spiritual community

Sanskrit: Ancient language used to write the Vedas, in chanting worship, and for mantras

Sat-chit-ananda: Being-consciousness-bliss

Satsang: Questions of a spiritual nature and answers from a Guru or acharya (spiritual teacher)

Shakti: Spiritual energy, especially associated with meditation and chanting; considered to be the active feminine aspect of the divine

SHAMBHAVANANDA: Great Kundalini meditation master and founder of the Shambhava School of Yoga

SHAMBHAVA YOGA: Hatha yoga with inner focus and attention to the breath; meditation practices following Kashmir Saivist principles and providing practical tools to bring spiritual practice into daily activities

SHAMBHAVI MUDRA: Remaining immersed in the consciousness of the inner Self while engaged in life's daily activities

SHIVA: Lord of destruction; one of the Hindu trinity of Brahma, Vishnu, and Shiva. Destroying the ego, Shiva reveals the universal consciousness within all.

SHANKARA: The meditative form of Shiva with the Ganges river flowing from his hair

SIDDHAS: Perfected beings

SIDDHIS: Extraordinary spiritual powers

SUBTLE BODY: The energetic body in which the dream state occurs

SUSHUMNA: Main energy channel corresponding to the spine

TAPASYA: Discipline and spiritual practices that heat and purify

TEMPLE: Spiritual place of worship where the three worlds of the humans, deities, and enlightened masters come together

TENSION RELEASE EXERCISE: Pranayama exercise to release negative psychic tensions

VEDAS: Ancient authorative Hindu texts from India

VISHNU: Lord of preservation. One of the Hindu trinity of Brahma, Vishnu, and Shiva.

VISUDDHA: Fourth chakra; spiritual energy center located at the throat

YAJNA: Fire ceremony using yantra, mantra, and rice masala offerings; conducted to establish harmonious vibrations in the atmosphere, people, and region

YOGA: Union of the body, breath, and mind

YOGACHARYA: Honorific title for an advanced yoga teacher

Bibliography

Brown, Christina. *The Yoga Bible.* Hampshire, UK, Godsfield Press Ltd., 2003.

Desikachar, T.K.V. *The Heart of Yoga: Developing a Personal Practice.* Rochester, Vermont, Inner Traditions Intl., 1999.

Frawley, David. *Yoga and Ayurveda: Self-Healing and Self-Realization.* Twin Lakes, WI, Lotus Press, 1999.

Iyengar, B.K.S. *Light on Pranayama: The Yogic Art of Breathing.* New York, NY, The Crossroads Publishing Company, 2000.

Iyengar, B.K.S. *Light on Yoga.* New York, NT, Schocker Books Inc., 1979.

Ma Yogashakti Saraswati, Maha Mandaleshwar, *Simplified Yogasanas & Pranayams*

Pandit, Bansi. *The Hindu Mind.* Glen Ellyn, IL, B & V Enterprises, Inc., 1998.

Shambhavananda, Sri. *A Seat by the Fire.* Rollinsville, CO, Prakasha Press, 2005.

Shambhavananda, Swami. *Spontaneous Recognition.* Eldorado Springs, CO SGRY, 1995.

Stone, Faith. *Rudi and the Green Apple.* Rollinsville, CO, SGRY, 2000.

Index

Page references for illustrations/sidebars and the names of postures are in italicized typeface. Terms, including glossary terms, appear in boldface.

With her fun and light-hearted teaching style, yogacharya Swami Omkari Devananda has led over 1,000 students in 200- and 500-hour yoga teacher training programs at the Shambhava School. She met Sri Shambhavananda while completing her degree in atmospheric chemistry at the University of Colorado. A student of his for 27 years, she has led hatha yoga workshops across the mainland United States, in Hawaii, and also in Tokyo. She has four published DVDs on beginner, intermediate, back care, and chair yoga.

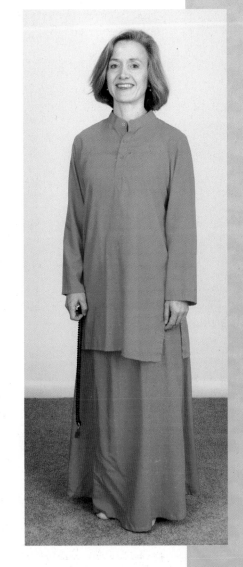

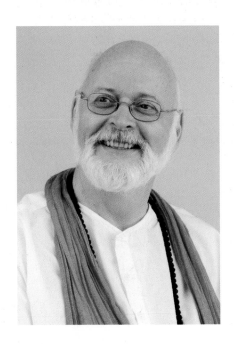

Bob Carter, graphic designer and owner of Blue Fusion Design, has had many opportunities to do photography for magazines. His passion, however, is to do photo shoots for vedic rituals, fire ceremonies, and Hindu temple celebrations. His work here, photographing hatha yoga postures, shows his versatility at catching the yogic sparkle in each model.

BOOK PUBLISHING COMPANY

since 1974—books that educate, inspire, and empower

To find your favorite vegetarian and soyfood products
online, visit: www.healthy-eating.com

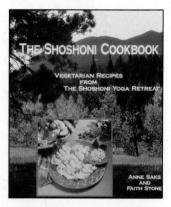

The Shoshoni Cookbook
Anne Saks and Faith Stone
978-0-913990-49-3
$14.95

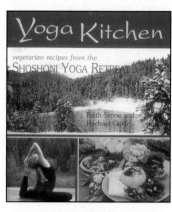

Yoga Kitchen
Faith Stone and Rachael Guidry
978-1-57067-145-6
$18.95

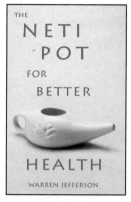

**The Neti Pot for Better
Health**
Warren Jefferson
978-1-57067-186-9
$9.95

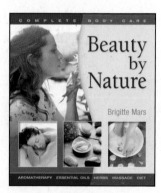

Beauty by Nature
Brigitte Mars
978-1-57067-193-7
$19.95

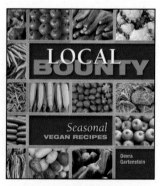

Local Bounty
Devra Gartenstein
978-1-57067-219-4
$17.95

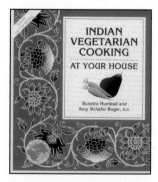

**Indian Vegetarian Cooking at
Your House**
Sunetra Humbad and Amy Schafer
Boger, MD
978-1-57067-004-6
$14.95

Purchase these health titles and cookbooks from your local bookstore or
natural food store, or you can buy them directly from:
Book Publishing Company • P.O. Box 99 • Summertown, TN 38483 • 1-800-695-2241
Please include $3.95 per item for shipping and handling.